Praise for H. Kenneth Fisher MD

Several books have been written on the subject of sleep: some for the general public and some are mostly scientific. This book by Dr. Ken Fisher has something for everyone. The book is an easy read, is delightfully concise, and gives you the feeling that he is talking directly to you.

JD Hudson, MD
Diplomate, American Board of Sleep Medicine
Fellow, American Board of Neurology

This comprehensive book is a timely reflection, written by a passionate physician with a keen interest in sleep who explores all aspects of this essential part of our lives. ... With a blend of medical expertise, personal anecdotes, and advice it provides readers with the deeper understanding of sleep that will stand them in good stead in the coming years. This is a book that is needed in all home libraries.

Adrian Williams, FRCP, FAASM
Consultant Physician and Professor of Sleep Medicine
King's College London.
Chief Medical Advisor
Circadian Health.
Past Clinical Director
Sleep Disorders Centre, Guy's and St Thomas, London.

With *Sleep: A User's Guide,* Dr. Ken Fisher takes the reader on an immersive journey into the fascinating world of slumber. As a sleep medicine specialist, he sheds light on common nocturnal disorders and offers the readers valuable insights to help understand and manage sleep concerns. Bravo, Dr. Fisher, for providing an exceptional resource for professionals and for the rest of us.

William Solberg DDS,
UCLA Professor of Dentistry, retired.

Sleep: A User's Guide is a slim but mighty volume. In a conversational style that is both easy-to-read and understandable, Dr. Fisher has given us a work that will be useful to all: young or old, man or woman, patient or professional. ... If you are not satisfied with the way you feel, allow Dr. Fisher to lead you along a path that is understandable and easy to follow. ... Overall, reading this book will give you a better understanding of the Hows and Whys of sleep. *Sleep: A User's Guide* is a fascinating read.

David Meltzer, MD
Diplomate of the American Board of Psychiatry and Neurology

Dr. Fisher writes clearly, from two perspectives: easy-to-follow discussions of common sleep problems, and plain language explanations of fascinating research studies. Both help us understand the wide-ranging connections between our own sleep and its effect on every part of our body. *Sleep: A Users Guide* is a significant resource for everyone.

Anson J Levine, PhD
Jungian Analyst

This book is a must-read for anyone who has a desire to operate at peak potential with a good quality of life. As *Sleep: A User's Guide* illustrates, lack of sleep increases the brain's tendency towards anger, and the entire body's risk of diabetes, obesity and generally poor performance. Due to the rise in school anger-related incidents and phone-use addiction, *Sleep: A User's Guide* will be of special interest to educators, students and athletes.

Adrian Baer, MA Ed.

SLEEP

sleep
A User's Guide

H. Kenneth Fisher MD

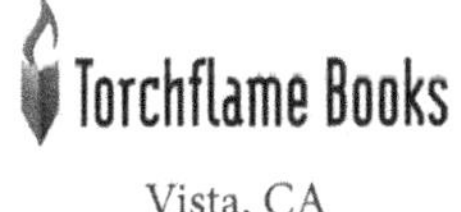

Vista, CA

ISBN: 978-1-61153-580-8 (paperback)

ISBN: 978-1-61153-581-5 (ebook)

ISBN: 978-1-61153-596-9 (large print)

Library of Congress Control Number: 2024919882

Sleep: A User's Guide is published by: Torchflame Books, an imprint of Top Reads Publishing, LLC, 1035 E. Vista Way, Suite 205, Vista, CA 92084, USA

For information about special discounts for bulk purchases, please direct emails to: publisher@torchflamebooks.com

Cover design and interior layout: Jori Hanna

Contents

This book is dedicated to the memory of my parents, Besse A. Fisher and Harry E. Fisher, and to Judith Roedelheimer Pacht, without whom the fall season of my life would likely have been experienced as winter.

Preface

Literally tens of millions of our fellow Americans and many millions more overseas suffer from sleep disorders: most commonly they "can't sleep," or they feel sleepy when they expect to be wide awake, or else have some disturbing form of physical activity that interrupts their sleep. This book will help victims of sleep disorders understand what causes the problems they face and how they can get better, more reliable sleep: the activity that usefully occupies one-third of their lives.

During recent years, startling new discoveries have shown how this complicated, enormously important part of our lives actually works in each person's body. Scientists can now see which cells in our brains talk to each other when we dream. As you gain a deeper understanding of your own sleep, I hope you will have less anxiety about differences you may notice between your own sleep and the sleep of others you know. A reader can choose among many books to answer his or her questions about sleep, but this book will be of special interest to all who are students at any age because healthy sleep is essential to learning of every kind. As people everywhere continue to live longer lives, there will be many millions who must work longer years to support themselves in their longer years of retirement—and so will need to continue learning well past the traditional "student years" of youth.

This book is written from the viewpoint of a practicing physician. My reasons for writing it are three. First, as a practicing medical doctor I have gradually learned that people feel more comfortable when they understand the health problems they face. It took years for the realization to hit me that my main responsibility was not just to make a clever diagnosis: it was always more important to reassure my patients that help was available in nearly every case and to explain what that help might look like. (I offer sincere apologies to my early patients.) This book is written in that spirit. Second, I am by nature and career a teacher. It's my pleasure when I can help people understand things that they may find puzzling, weird, or obscure. Third, I simply love understanding the mysteries of nature. When I can help others join me in that excitement, I'm having a great day.

So, I invite you to come along with me as we explore "the symphony of sleep" and see how our sleep is organized. Then we'll get an overview of the many things that can produce less-than-perfect sleep; and finally we'll take a look at the wider significance of sleep and its disturbances. We'll see how this genius of a body we each have manages the faint electrical signals within different parts of our brain and in the rest of our body to make it all happen—usually with musical precision. At every turn, we'll make clear what you can do to improve your own sleep when it's less than perfectly satisfying.

Many friends and colleagues have offered suggestions for

improving this book, but full responsibility for all errors and shortcomings is my own.

H. Kenneth Fisher MD
Los Angeles

1

The Overture to Sleep (and how this book can help you)

Large numbers of people just like us feel they waste too much time sleeping, yearn to sleep better, wish they weren't feeling sleepy so much of the time, or wonder why their sleep sometimes seems bizarre. If you are among them, or even if you would just like to better understand, enjoy, and appreciate the bargain value of spending roughly one-third of your life asleep—then this book is for you.

No matter what your personal sleep issues are, a good place to start is by recognizing that consistency of sleep habits is important. To my own patients, I have usually recommended they decide what is the earliest time they must get out of bed during their typical week's schedule. Make that the time to get up every single day, and allow for one "late or lazy" day each week if you so choose. Set an alarm for that same wake-up time daily, so there's no temptation to frequently check the clock. (Doing so can get your anxiety turned on, and that doesn't help your sleep.) Do get up when the alarm goes off, as that helps anchor your own body clock rhythms. Exposure to bright light at that time further helps set your body clock to match society's daily demands.

Deciding when to turn off the lights for sleep is now a matter of counting backwards for the number of hours that makes you feel best. For most people, the length of their natural sleep period is a little longer than eight hours. Yours may be different—even several hours longer or shorter. If you feel rested and well with that different amount, you'll probably do just fine to stick with what works best for you. If you do not feel rested and even a week or two with eight hours a night in bed for sleep doesn't make you feel well rested, it's time to consult a sleep specialist.

Sleep has been surprisingly popular as long as there's been life on Earth. Even one-celled creatures such as bacteria, if they live longer than one day, have periods of rest alternating with periods of activity. Invertebrates (organisms too primitive to have a spinal cord) sleep, and they've been on Earth for more than five hundred million years. Fish sleep. Birds sleep, even while they're in full flight during migrations of thousands of miles, even over open ocean. Their trick is that one-half of their brain sleeps at a time, and the two sides take turns. Every animal we know sleeps, even though for nearly all of them, that's risky: they aren't as aware of possible danger and aren't fully ready to run or fight for their lives. It's no accident that many predators are active mainly during the night, when their prey sleep.

Newborn human babies act as if sleep is not a waste of their time. They spend up to twenty hours a day sleeping. The only other thing worth their time, it seems, is feeding. Why aren't they busy learning to talk, to crawl, or something more useful than "just" sleeping?

Many (if not all) plants sleep. You may be familiar with the closing up of the flowers of certain plants at night and their reopening for business with the reappearance of daylight.[1] In reality, some reopen at the right time even without light.[2]

If you have more than a few days of trouble falling asleep or staying asleep, it's time to check out a book mentioned in chapter 9: *No More Sleepless Nights* by (the late) Peter Hauri and Shirley Linde. That book helps you review all the factors in your own life that can help—or interfere—with routinely satisfying and restorative sleep. If you still need help after that, try the references in chapter 9 to in-person or online self-directed CBT-I (cognitive behavioral therapy for insomnia). Most sleep clinics and many MDs and other psychotherapists offer personalized CBT-I for help with chronic insomnia.

For those with troublesome levels of sleepiness, the path to improvement starts with assuring that you do have enough time in bed for your sleep needs. Despite what's become common in our culture, most of us really do need about eight hours a night for sleep. If you have that and are still sleepier than you think you should be, it's time to try your hand at being Sherlock Holmes. Can you identify any factors that could be disturbing your sleep hours? Are you snoring? Do you have leg or arm movements in your sleep? (You may need help from a bed partner to identify some of these problems, as they may occur only when you're too deeply asleep to be aware of them.) Do you often stop breathing during the night? Even if these problems seem infrequent to you and you're not aware of them arousing you during the night, you'll need professional help from a sleep specialist to check them out. Do you have sleep "attacks" that are overwhelming during the day? That's an automatic "time out!" to see a sleep specialist. The same is true of cataplexy: the occasional and abrupt involuntary relaxation of muscles that leads to dropping things as different as your coffee, your eyelids, or your entire body without losing consciousness. Treatment for excessive daytime sleepiness varies, depending on the condition. For obstructive sleep apnea —affecting dozens of millions in the US alone—you could try avoiding sleep in the supine position—i.e. don't sleep flat on your back. In some (less severe) sleep apnea patients, that can sometimes solve the problem. Most will need formal evaluation and some more complex form of treatment. The most widely used currently is CPAP (continuous positive airway pressure) applied with a face mask during sleep. Other methods of treatment are mentioned in chapter 10.

What about repeated limb movements during the night? If cutting way back on caffeine doesn't fix or at least greatly improve the problem, help from a specialist is probably needed. They will likely order an overnight sleep study and possibly one or more blood tests to check your body's iron supply.

If you are troubled by other unexpected or odd behaviors during the night, you will be served best by bringing to a sleep specialist all the information you can to describe the troubling behavior. Both falling asleep and waking up bring very large changes in the electrical and chemical background in the brain, and unusual experiences can occur, especially at those times. Examples include being awake but unable to move (known as sleep paralysis, usually lasting only a few minutes) and actual hallucinations. Some of these can initially be very frightening, but reassurance usually comes with a diagnosis and treatment.

Given all that popularity, you might well ask, "Why is sleep so important?" What is going on during the hours of sleep that makes it such a high priority that we're willing to take the risk of being off-guard in the dark, night after night, instead of being at our desks, catching supper, or playing video games?

For us, sleep is especially—but not only—an activity of the brain. There is evidence in humans that every cell in the body has a cycle of activity that includes keeping time with our internal sleep-regulating clock(s). Sleepiness also appears to be a matter of chemistry. Early in the twentieth century, Henri Pieron found that if he transferred spinal fluid from sleep-deprived dogs into the spinal fluid space of other dogs, the recipient dogs also became sleepy.[3]

Sleep is one of four basic drives to behavior: the drives to eat, drink, reproduce, and sleep. But a single night without sleep brings far more trouble than a night without any of the other three. As we will see in some detail later, adequate sleep has very important benefits for learning and memory (chapter 5), physical performance and skill (chapter 7), creativity (chapter 8), and emotional stability (chapter 9). Increasing awareness of the value of sleep has led athletes, their coaches, and numerous creative organizations to make special arrangements to ensure their prized personnel get the benefits of adequate sleep. Military intelligence officers wanting to intimidate their captives into cooperation, unfortunately, sometimes use sleep deprivation as a form of enhanced interrogation.

Most of us dream every night, but not all of us are aware of our dreams or remember many of them. If yours are especially frightening or repeatedly bizarre, it's worth seeking help from a psychotherapist or sleep specialist. How dreams occur, and some insight into their significance are described in chapter 6.

Our sleep is closely related to our mental health. If you are prone to depression or think you may be bipolar, it's important to be on the lookout for worsening sleep. That's a time to get help without delay to avoid a downward spiral of both sleep and mental health. Self-help is probably not the best first step in that situation. Therapists can recommend ways to combat severe depression and help you avoid sleep-related episodes of bipolar disorder.

What about other unusual experiences you're having with your sleep? They may seem less mysterious when we remember that different parts of the brain can actually be (at the same time) in stages of sleep that are different from each other. You will meet a woman in chapter 11 who could not remember how she had fractured her pelvis during the previous night's sleep. She was almost certainly in deep sleep in part of her brain, yet clearly awake enough elsewhere in her brain to leave bed and fall hard enough to sustain a major fracture—without even waking up. She then found her way back to bed for the rest of the night—again without waking up. For anything resembling this kind of puzzling experience, professional help is needed.

When scientists study sleep, they find patterns that recur at roughly predictable intervals during the night. Typically, roughly every ninety minutes of sleep, we have a new series of nerve cell electrical signals, with recognizable patterns reoccurring—something like the movements of a symphony. These shorter patterns (movements) are described by the sleep stages discussed in chapter 2. Because these recurring patterns (detected on the scalp during overnight sleep studies) resemble the movements of symphonic music and the recurring musical themes the movements contain, I like to use the term "symphony of sleep" to draw attention to the similarities between a night's sleep and a typical symphony.

Whatever is your reason for taking the time to read this book, the increasingly wide interest in learning about sleep means you're in good company. The public's interest in sleep has grown as lots more usable information has become available about this complicated and highly organized part of our lives. Whatever problems you may have with your own sleep, you can feel assured that well-trained men and women are available all over this country (and in much of the world) to help you with proven and effective treatments for most of the more than one hundred known sleep disorders.

2

What's Happening in the Brain When We Sleep?

For most of history, sleep was viewed simply as a turning-off of the body and mind. Everybody knew it was important, but no one had any idea why. Shakespeare recognized sleep's healing property: "Sleep, that knits up the ravele'd sleeve of care." [1] Until almost the end of the nineteenth century, the world had learned very little about what happens during human sleep. That's changed a lot within the lifetime of our senior citizens.

During sleep, the brain's neurons are not quiet. Instead, there's constant "chatter" among them. When a brain cell (neuron) is turned on, it creates a tiny electrical signal. These tiny electrical signals pass from one neuron to another and are the basis of communication: information is being passed from one part of the brain to another. Sensitive instruments placed on the surface of the scalp about a hundred years ago showed that there are distinct patterns within these signals, and those patterns show up over and over again during every night of human sleep. These patterns make up the symphony of sleep.

There are several patterns, some occurring only once each

night. Others repeat roughly every ninety minutes during sleep. Within each ninety-minute cycle, there are additional patterns. At UCLA, Rechtschaffen and Kales[2] recognized and described some of these signal patterns. The characteristic pattern of stage 1 sleep usually appears after a period of drowsiness. The closed eyes move slowly back and forth, and characteristic "alpha" electrical waves are found, especially over the back of the head, as we become increasingly drowsy.

During stage 1 sleep, people can be awakened easily by noise. They can notice changes in the brightness of light and keep rough track of time without looking at any clock. They can also have reverie-type thoughts. (These features will be important when we discuss sleep stage misperception in chapter 9.) In adults, stage 1 sleep usually lasts only a few minutes just as sleep starts, and it's seen later on, briefly, and occasionally throughout the night.

Stage 2 sleep is seen during more of our sleep than any other stage (usually around half our sleep for adults). Against a background of the irregular and low-voltage signals of stage 1, stage 2 sleep also includes occasional high-voltage but slow discharge patterns (called K-complexes) and brief bursts of low-voltage, fast discharges (called sleep spindles).

As we'll see, modern imaging technology has helped us learn a lot about the role these signal patterns play in creating and processing our memories. It's harder to wake someone from stage 2 sleep than from stage 1.[3] During stage 2 sleep, we can't keep track of time, and we have no more dreamy thoughts.

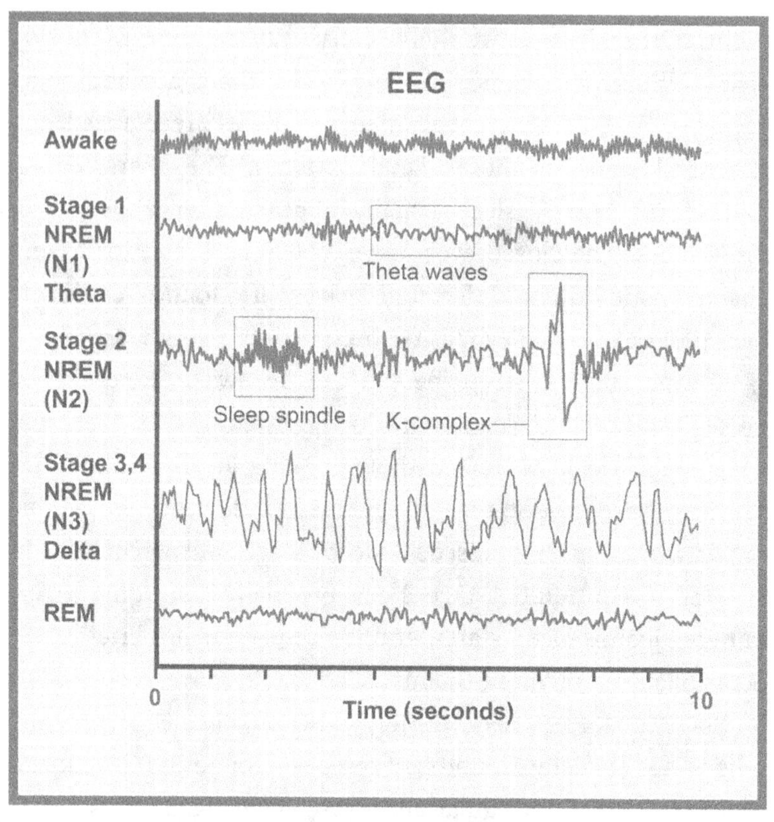

Credit to Cordelia Molloy / Science Photo Library

Delta sleep (stages 3 and 4) is astonishingly different. There, the high-voltage (and slow) electrical waves we see mean that lots of neurons beneath the scalp detectors are firing, nearly in lockstep with each other. These successive tsunami waves of electrical signals move from the forehead straight toward the back of the head. This is a big contrast to the scattered signals that form the background of the wake state, and of stage 1 sleep, stage 2 sleep, and even stage REM (which we'll discuss later in this chapter). These very different electrical signal patterns of the different stages of sleep suggest that very different neurological events are taking place within our brains during these different sleep stages.

During childhood, we gradually spend more and more of our sleep in very deep (delta) sleep, reaching a maximum just before puberty. Delta sleep seems to support the disconnection of neurologic circuits that are no longer needed. If we don't prune these brain circuits enough (as can happen with abnormal delta sleep), we are at risk of developing schizophrenia.[4]

After age thirty, the amount of delta sleep slips down from a high point of about 20 percent of our sleep time to almost none by age seventy. The loss of delta sleep isn't the same everywhere in the brain: it moves from the back of the head toward the front. As this change gradually plays out, we steadily lose some of our ability to retain new learning overnight. As a result, older adults typically retain overnight only half as much new information as younger adults.

In some senses, delta sleep is the deepest form of sleep. It's very hard to wake anyone up from this state. Scientists think that's because the chemical and nerve cell environment within the brain lasts for several minutes after arousal from delta sleep. That's very different from waking up from stage REM sleep—when, within ninety seconds, the brain's chemical environment has usually gone right back to the normal awake state. This slowness to awaken from delta sleep gives rise to the phenomenon of sleep inertia. Disorders (such as night terrors, seen especially in young children) that start from delta sleep often produce confusion along with very little conscious awareness of the surroundings. Surprisingly, the victim can usually still navigate his way around the bedroom with no difficulty.

Modern imaging has helped us understand a lot of what happens during delta sleep, especially how we process memories. Sleep scientists have found that increasing the amount of delta sleep brings improved overnight memory for new information. To make that happen experimentally and safely, Swiss sleep scientists recently showed that it's not only infants who can be helped into sleep by a gentle rocking motion. They showed that healthy adults, too, fell asleep faster in a gently rocking bed; they also had more delta sleep and had better recall for new memories the next morning.[5] This surprising result tells us that during sleep—even though the brain loses conscious awareness of an external factor like a rocking bed—that same brain is still greatly influenced by the rocking motion. This was made clear by the appearance of more highly synchronized waves of delta sleep in the brains of the rocking bed volunteers and by their improved memory.

Stage REM is considered by some experts to be so different from both wakefulness and each of the sleep stages described so far that it represents a totally different state of being. It is a state of very high metabolic activity in the brain: our brains use more oxygen per minute during stage REM than they do even during full wakefulness. The baseline electrical signals over the scalp during stage REM are like those of wakefulness and stages 1 and 2: that is, low voltage, fast, seemingly randomly irregular firing of nerve cells "chattering" beneath the scalp. What is highly unusual during stage REM is the characteristic rapid, coordinated (typically side-to-side), alternating eye movements, with the total paralysis of nearly all voluntary muscles (the ones that we're usually able to control).

During life in the womb, REM-like activity plays an important role in the brain's development. During the second and third trimesters of pregnancy, the amount of stage REM (or the very similar electrical activity pattern investigators can see in that immature brain) increases quickly and reaches about half the baby's total sleep time in the final week before full-term birth at thirty-eight weeks of gestation. Never again will the brain spend this much of its time in stage REM. (Usually, stage REM takes up about 20 percent of the night's sleep in healthy adults.) Even so, newborn infants can't seem to get enough. They don't even show any other kind of sleep pattern until age two or three months.[6] While we don't yet know all the tasks that keep the infant brain so busy during this time, it is known from animal studies that the developing fetal brain shows very active coating of nerve cell fibers (axons) with insulating sheaths made up of myelin, a fatty material.[7] We would expect that an individual nerve fiber, once insulated that way, could transmit an electrical signal down its entire length without disturbing the neighboring nerve fibers. This would allow each nerve fiber to belong to one or more specialized collections of neurons called circuits.

Circuits made up of myelin-insulated neurons could act quite independently of other nerve fibers and other circuits, even those found right next door. We can speculate that the intense metabolic activity found in the brain of the fetus is needed to prepare that brain for the coming development of individual brain circuits. Many new circuits will soon be needed for the learning tasks of infancy and early childhood. If anything interferes with the REM-requiring period of creating new synapses and circuits, there can be disastrous consequences. For now, though, the importance of sufficient REM can stand alone: children who have insufficient REM during early development of the brain can be faced with major disorders: those with autism, for example, have 30 percent less REM than normal.[8] As we've noted, later on in infancy and early childhood, during delta sleep, the brain is busy pruning away electrical circuits that are no longer needed.

Stage REM was unknown until the middle of the last century. For its discovery, we owe thanks to Aserinsky and Kleitman. Around 1953, at the University of Chicago, they noticed that sleeping cats and dogs sometimes showed abrupt running movements with sudden changes in their brain's electrical activity.[9] The animals also started showing rapid back-and-forth eye movements, even though they appeared to be fully asleep. They called this rapid eye movement or REM sleep, and similar observations were soon made in human infants.[10] It's now known that stage REM is a period rich in dreams. Although the behavior changes just mentioned are unique to stage REM, changes in various body functions are also seen with shifts among the other sleep stages described by Rechtschaffen and Kales. These include changes in breathing, heartbeat, muscle tone, and sensitivity to altered blood levels of oxygen and carbon dioxide (that occur as we breathe more shallowly or more deeply).

Although a lot is known about what happens throughout the body during sleep, there are still many mysteries to unravel —especially within the brain. Of course, it should be no surprise that we don't completely understand how the brain works. After all, as Burnett observed, "If the human brain were so simple that we could understand it, we would be so simple that we couldn't."[11]

3

How Long Do We Really Need for Sleep?

One way of learning the importance of sleep is to see what happens without enough of it. Isn't it striking, for example, how easily lectures and church sermons become boring when we're very sleepy? We all know how hard it is to pay attention at those times. Focusing our attention is clearly one of the many things that doesn't work well when we're sleep-deprived. Unfortunately, that shows up in news reports of car crashes, navigational errors (Exxon Valdez), judgment errors (Three Mile Island), and disasters elsewhere (Chernobyl). In each of these widely reported cases, there was evidence that those responsible for the accidents were working in a sleep-deprived state. When the Exxon Valdez ran aground in Alaskan waters, for example, it was being piloted by the third mate, who was severely sleep-deprived. He had been working long hours for several days with no sleep in the hours leading up to the accident.

Leaving for a moment the question of how much sleep is enough, we can all agree that when we don't get enough sleep, we know there's something wrong. If we don't get enough sleep during the workweek, we feel better after "catching up" on the weekends. However, every student may as well learn right now that the damage to week-day learning caused by losses of sleep during the weekdays can never be overcome by weekend catch-up sleep.

Not only do we feel better when we're adequately rested, but we do much better on tests of both brain and physical performance. Using tests of mistakes in simple arithmetic, driving control, word recall, or athletic performance, studies have shown that a single night without sleep causes as many errors as being legally drunk.[1] By the way, the legal blood alcohol standard for being drunk varies among nations: the UK's standard for intoxication is lower than the United States' standard, and Norway's is much lower. Sleep deprivation causes as many errors as a blood alcohol level meeting the American standard for intoxication, which puts it far beyond acceptable by any measure.

Professor Jerry Siegel at UCLA has studied three separate pre-industrial societies. He explains how they showed similar sleep patterns in very different geographic locations and cultures.

People tend to get up around daybreak and go back to sleep about seven to nine hours before the next dawn. However, this pattern can vary as the seasons change.

During the past one hundred years, the average night's sleep in this country has shrunk by about a full hour.[2] That gradual change is due to greater access to electricity, light bulbs, and entertainment brought into the home by radio, television, and the internet. In addition, work demands are changing through shift work and international business activity across multiple time zones. Besides that, there's the increased work of women who often have an outside job in addition to the job of being the major homemaker. There's no evidence that the average human brain has changed over this time period, so we are either getting less sleep than we need or we were previously getting too much sleep. Various studies indicate that, on average, American adults get fewer than seven hours of sleep per night now, as opposed to eight hours each night a century ago. Forty percent of us get fewer than six hours a night.[3,4] Would you expect that decreased sleep to come at a cost?

An early approach to the question of sleep needs was made by two scientists who slept in a cave for a month, totally isolated from the normal cues of sunlight and the activities of the society around them. Each man slept, on average, more than eight hours a night, though their individual averages weren't the same.[5]

To learn if our society's habits produce a "sleep debt," investigators at the US Naval Hospital in Bethesda, Maryland, asked a number of healthy young adult volunteers to stay in bed twenty-four hours a day in a darkened and soundproof room every day for a whole week. Every extra hour they slept beyond eight hours every twenty-four hours was counted as an hour of "residual sleep debt." The main result was an astonishing average of twenty-five extra hours of sleep during that one week.[6] These results have been confirmed by other sleep studies. Either our bodies are simply greedy for sleep, or we are far more sleep deprived as a society than most of us recognize. Remembering that sleep has been such a risky behavior for most of human history, we might suspect the second possibility is the real one.

Some people claim to be perfectly healthy and wide awake with less sleep than others need. There is evidence that such short-sleepers do exist and can flourish. There is an inherited basis for this pattern[7] in some individuals, but others who make the same claim may be fooling themselves. The great inventor Thomas Edison reportedly slept only four hours at night, but he frequently took short naps—or, as we might popularly call them today, power naps. It's been shown that even ten minutes of uninterrupted sleep is enough to restore alertness temporarily in a sleepy person. In my practice, I've worked with several patients that serve as living proof of the clinical research reported here. To begin, one which illustrates the importance of even short bursts of sleep for brain function:

A twenty-seven-year-old man drove alone from California to St. Louis to meet a deadline. After a two-thousand-mile trip with little sleep time, he reached the target city around 5 a.m. on a beautiful, clear summer day. Increasingly, he was struggling to stay awake and keep the car on the road, even when he was less than five miles from home. It occurred to him that if he did not stop to sleep, he would probably not survive the last five miles. Pulling the car to the curb, he dozed for about fifteen minutes and was then able to proceed home safely.

Less than enough sleep is very expensive. Whatever the ideal amount of time for human sleep, the results of shortchanging our sleep needs are striking. If we compare the risk of motor vehicle accidents with the average hours of sleep (estimated by the drivers), we see a disturbing and very clear pattern: less sleep, more accidents.

A similar conclusion was reached in a study of driving simulators and sleep deprivation. Compared with well-rested participants who rarely drove off the road, those with one night of only four hours of sleep drove the simulator off-road six times as often. Those who became legally drunk and also had only four hours of sleep were thirty times as likely to steer off the road! To understand how that might happen, David Dinges at the University of Pennsylvania measured the number of microsleeps (each only a few seconds long) in subjects deprived of sleep. After one night with no sleep at all, there were four times as many microsleeps. Even with six hours of sleep each night for several nights, there was a steady increase in the number of micro-sleeps, reaching the same four-times increase after ten days.[8,]

The belief that frequent microsleeps imply a lower quality of sleep has recently been challenged, however, by surprising findings in the chinstrap penguins of the Antarctic region. Investigators headed by Paul-Antoine Libourel (of the Lyon Neuroscience Research Centre) have found no lengthy uninterrupted sleep in that species: the chinstrap penguins have as many as ten thousand microsleeps a day, lasting only four seconds or less each.[9]

How many of the drivers you'll pass driving today have had less than six hours of sleep most nights during this past week? How many hours of sleep, on average, will you have had?

If we look at length of life plotted against average hours of sleep, we see another hint that sleep pays off. An average sleep duration of less than seven hours a night is associated with greater mortality in both men and (even more in) women.[10] Full disclosure: the numbers supporting this statement also show that for average sleep time longer than nine hours per night, mortality begins to increase again. The significance of this information is debated: some of the people who sleep longer hours may have serious illness, which itself leads to early death. That might make us believe (incorrectly) that the longer sleep hours were the *cause* of the increased mortality. At this point, we honestly can't be sure and are unlikely to see an experimental study to find the truth. Personally, I'm not worried about healthy people who choose to sleep longer than eight hours a night.

Sleep deprivation studies have shown many harmful effects. These include mental effects: irritability, impaired ability to think, lapses of memory, impaired moral judgment, and hallucinations. Some symptoms may be confused with ADHD. There is increased heart rate variability and increased risk of heart disease. Muscle reaction time is slowed, and there are tremors, muscle aches, and decreased accuracy. There is an increased risk of type 2 diabetes and obesity. In youth, there is growth suppression.

During the years of my hospital residency, it was not uncommon for young physicians to go without sleep for nearly an entire night—or even a whole night—and then have another on-call night two days later after only one night off-call. After a period of several such alternating nights with little sleep, I found myself hallucinating and writing absolute gibberish into the medical record of a young woman whose exam I had just finished. Fortunately, medical residents no longer undergo such trials by fire, but the effects on older physicians—who for a number of years were left to deal with urgent middle-of-the-night problems of their own hospitalized patients—were largely ignored. Fortunately, this problem is now sometimes managed through the use of physicians specifically assigned to cover night calls (nocturnists).

The outcome of such sleep deprivation can be frightening. Published studies connected medical errors to long work hours and sleep deprivation, so the Council for Graduate Medical Education issued rules limiting weekly work hours and demanding minimal allowances for sleep. Residents after that were less depressed, but results were otherwise not very encouraging.[11]

Modern imaging technology has allowed scientists to see what changes in the brain's metabolic activity might cause these large effects on our health and our ability to function when short of sleep. As increasing numbers of us look forward to a longer lifespan, we also have to think about the need for periodically re-educating ourselves for new kinds of work. That means that the harmful effects of sleep loss on our ability to learn how to do new work will become more and more important. As noted earlier, after a single night without sleep, there's a 40 percent drop in the ability to learn new facts the next day. (Attention all students: so much for the value of all-nighters!)

Brain Structures Related to Sleep and Learning

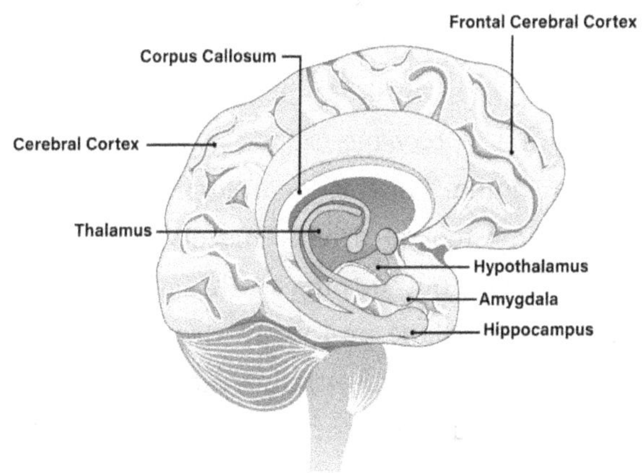

Retention and later recall are also severely impaired by sleep loss. An MRI (magnetic resonance images) after a night completely without sleep showed absolutely no metabolic activity in the hippocampus, the place where new information typically enters the brain. Think also for a moment about the amygdala, the brain's center for anger. After one night without sleep, functional brain MRIs show a 60 percent increase in activity of the amygdala. At the same time, the prefrontal cortex becomes electrically isolated from the amygdala, thus bringing decreased restraint by the brain's judgment center on the anger center. In this way, sleep loss effects might help explain the tendency of some sleep-deprived young adults to engage in behaviors they know are risky and to make bad quick decisions. If these occur behind the wheel, they can be—and too often are—lethal.

It's worth remembering that the auto insurance industry considers young male adults to be the most accident-prone drivers. The industry has the most detailed individual driver records available anywhere.

The combination of sleep deprivation with alcohol is especially dangerous. After several nights of Christmas holiday revelry with limited sleep, an eighteen-year-old youth stayed at a New Year's Eve party until 3 a.m. He was drinking so much alcohol that his fellow teenage friends pleaded with him to let them drive him home. However, confident that he was "perfectly okay" he insisted on driving his own car. Shortly after leaving the party without turning on his car's headlights, he entered a divided four-lane motorway, driving the wrong way, directly against the oncoming traffic. He drove head-on into another car carrying a family of four on their way home. He was the only survivor.

During the formative years of a child's development, there are other hints of profound damage from lack of adequate sleep. In the past few decades, there's been a large increase in the number of children (and adults) diagnosed with attention deficit disorder (ADD). The most popular and effective form of treatment for ADD involves the use of alerting medications, such as methylphenidate. These can bring remarkable benefits, but they can also interfere with sleep. In addition, other undesirable consequences have appeared in youth given Concerta (also methylphenidate). Volunteer subjects given Concerta tended to view photographs of facial expressions as significantly more hostile than did control subjects who were not given Concerta—raising anxiety over how this might affect the social behavior of those taking Concerta. This would be of increased concern when sleep deprivation has also increased activity in the amygdala, the center for anger.

It may soon become possible to reliably measure whether a child is getting enough sleep. Researchers Iacomino and colleagues have recently reported that blood levels of two different micro-RNA molecules showed good correlation with hours of sleep in more than one hundred children from different parts of Europe.[12]

Further, as we will explore in greater detail (in chapter 12), the relationship of inadequate sleep to excess weight, diabetes, hypertension, and obesity have a close link. The normal pattern is that during sleep, there is a dramatic increase in blood levels of leptin, a hormone thought to help us avoid feeling hunger, especially during the night. [13] An absence of hunger thus normally continues while we sleep. The dramatic decline in hours of sleep in the United States during the last sixty years has been matched by an equally dramatic rise in obesity. The pattern seems to be less sleep = less leptin = less control of appetite and more obesity.

Another study of the appetite-related hormones leptin and ghrelin showed that after two days of sleep restricted to four or five hours per night, the hormonal balance shifted to reduce the satiety-signaling hormone leptin, and this was associated with an average daily increase of three hundred calories in food eaten. If continued, this could result in a weight gain of ten to fifteen pounds per year. During my clinical training in the early 1960s, very long workdays led many of us (residents) to eat four full meals per day. It seems possible—maybe even likely—that the common complaint of undesired weight gain during freshman year at college may be due at least in part to the sleep deprivation to which many students unwisely subject themselves (as I did). Compounding the weight-control problem is this comparison: among dieters who sleep eight hours, half their weight loss comes from fat, whereas among dieters with fewer than six hours of sleep per night, 70 percent of their weight loss comes from muscle. This undesirable outcome is the price to be paid for dieting without enough sleep.[14]

When the yearly start of Daylight Savings Time shortens the sleep of millions of people by only one hour for only one night, there is a temporary but definite increase in the number of heart attacks. That pattern promptly returns to normal as the length of sleep does. (A group of sleep specialists is therefore trying to end the use of Daylight Savings Time altogether in the United States.) The immune system is also highly sensitive to sleep deprivation: one night of only four hours of sleep brings a 70 percent reduction in the number of natural killer T cells in the blood—the cells that help protect us against infection. Could this be why the best (and wholly natural) treatment for acute viral infections seems to be extra sleep? Astonishing increases in the power of molecular biology have shown how these many changes can be brought about by sleep loss. After one week of only six hours of sleep per night, investigators have found that more than seven hundred different genes show changes in the number of their product molecules made by transcription from their DNA.[15]

Intense research toward understanding and eventual control of Alzheimer's dementia has suggested the importance of build-up within the brain of the toxic protein beta-amyloid. Loss of delta sleep is associated with the accumulation of beta-amyloid in the medial frontal lobes of the brain. How might that happen? The mechanism seems to be that delta sleep brings a 60 percent shrinkage of glial cells within the brain. Since these cells line the channels used to flush waste out through the glymphatic system, their shrinkage (during delta sleep) leads to a widening of the channels and increased flushing. Both beta-amyloid and Tau protein (another naturally occurring brain toxin) are normally cleared this way, so that loss of delta sleep as we age beyond thirty years leads to a gradual accumulation of these toxic proteins. Sleep deprivation would further impair that vital clearance function. We'd better flush those toxins out while we can still produce delta sleep, before we are "timed out" by age.

One of the most disastrous effects of sleep deprivation is that we can no longer recognize how sleepy we have become. Awareness of sleepiness while driving is definitely not enough to prevent car crashes.[16]

So what determines when we get sleepy? There are two body systems at play. One is simply the clock: once we're in a stable sleep pattern day after day, we tend to get sleepy at the same time each day as our usual sleep time approaches. The clock that matters most is not the one on the table; it's the one inside our cells—probably every single cell in our body. Strangely, these (molecular) clocks tend to operate on a daily rhythm that's not the same as the Earth's twenty-four-hour daily cycle. Our Earth's day is based on our planet's rotation on its own axis and the resulting exposure to the sun. But our internal clocks usually have a cycle that's about fifteen to twenty minutes longer than the twenty-four-hour Earth day. If we are left alone, we'll be going to sleep later and later, as our "day" would end later and later compared with the clock on the table. Each of us has a "day" that is characteristic for us but may differ from other people's (as the investigators concluded from the cave experiments mentioned previously).

To some degree, we're rescued from that progressive delay in bedtime by our other way to get sleepy: the steady accumulation in our body of one or more chemicals that keep building up until we get to sleep and reduce them. The main chemical that provides that signal appears to be adenosine. The minute we wake up, that chemical starts building up again, only to be gradually flushed out whenever we fall asleep again.

A further check on our getting wildly out of phase with society around us is the community pressure insisting that we have a schedule to meet—at school, at work, for meals, for meetings, (for golf or tennis?)—and these stick with the timing of our mechanical clock on the table. Each day that we get up at our usual time helps reset us back from our longer-than-twenty-four-hour natural clock.

Think for a moment about the huge changes in our natural daily (circadian) rhythms as we go through different stages of our own lives. As infants, we're programmed to wake with the sun and fall asleep at an appropriate interval later, but by the time we're adolescents, we're tempted to avoid sleep during the night almost until the sun rises, and we have real trouble waking up early enough for school. By the time we reach old age, our personal circadian rhythms have shifted dramatically again. Then we may have trouble staying awake even in the early or mid-evening and also have trouble staying asleep until sunrise because our internal clocks tell us early that it's time to restart our personal day again.

The most powerful force of all, keeping us in tune with our environment, is exposure to morning sunlight. This "zeitgeber" (time-giver) of light exposure is maximal at around 9 a.m. (in the pre-modern societies studied by Siegel) and helps coordinate our internal rhythms of alertness every day with the world around us. In a later chapter, we'll see what happens when our internal clocks don't match our societal needs.

Military leaders have always sought ways to keep their soldiers awake longer, to gain an advantage over their enemies. During World War II, literally millions of German soldiers and civilians were encouraged to take Pervitin (the brand name for methamphetamine) pills to keep them alert and working for longer periods.[17] Recent evidence has shown the folly of this strategy, however. With increasing sleep deprivation inevitably comes increasing errors in judgment.

The big take-home message of this chapter is that to function normally, we humans need an average of about eight hours of sleep a night. There's some evidence that we can perform even better with more sleep than that. (Notice tennis champion Roger Federer's habit of sleeping several hours more, especially on the nights before important matches.)[18] It's likely, however, that most of us differ only a little from the average requirement of eight hours.

4

Your Body Has Clocks

A zoology professor told my undergraduate class about new studies of saltwater crabs and their amazing ability to keep time. When the tide came in to their native cove, the color of their carapace (shell) would change, right in time with the tide. But if they were moved overnight to a nearby cove (where the tide came in at a different time), it took them several days to adjust the timing of their color change to match the tides in the new location. They were keeping time overnight with their original cove. We humans sometimes have similar challenges.

A forty-year-old computer engineer and businessman was in excellent health but needed to fly from London to Southern California (home), and soon thereafter to Tokyo. In each place he needed to be alert enough to arrange business deals during the local business hours. If he were sleepy, he would risk making expensive mistakes. How could he stay as alert as possible without needing to stay in each city long enough to get acclimated to the local time zone? After reviewing the options together, we agreed to have him start his night-time sleep hours during each flight as soon as possible, and to use a sleeping medicine (Ambien) on the plane about half an hour before the desired bedtime at the new location. This seemed to be helpful, though not perfect. In retrospect, it might have been more helpful to use carefully timed melatonin supplementation instead of Ambien, as that might have helped reset his internal clocks rather than simply putting him to sleep at the desired time.

Marco Polo did not have this problem when he first traveled across seven or eight time zones from the Italian city of Venice to the eastern Chinese court of Kublai Khan in the thirteenth century. The trip took months, which allowed his internal clocks to adjust gradually to the daytime hours in each new location. For better or worse, we can now make the same journey in just a few hours, but our internal clocks simply can't cope with such fast changes. Without artificial help, we can adjust our internal clocks by about forty-five minutes each day when we travel east (to later time zones) and by about one hour each day when we travel west (to earlier time zones). Anyone who must attend early meetings in a new time zone may be forced to adjust quickly to the new daybreak but usually has a little more control over her lights-out time. Appropriate short-term use of melatonin or sleep aides like Ambien can be useful, but the timing of the medicine is important and should ideally be selected with the help of a sleep specialist.

An attorney brought his college junior son on a Friday for help about ten days before the son was scheduled to return to the University of California Berkeley for his final year. The son was afraid he'd be unable to adjust to morning classes. All summer, he'd been working as a disk jockey until 2 a.m. or later, and he did not get to sleep until 4 or 5 a.m. Then he would sleep until noon or later. I pointed out that the time remaining before school restarted was pretty short compared with the large change needed in sleeping habits. In any case, the son seemed unwilling to change his current habits at all. As I was personally scheduled to begin a long trip three days after the initial consultation, we couldn't arrange a follow-up visit before school was to start again. After making suggestions for the gradual readjustment of the student's sleeping schedule, I lost track of him. His father seemed unhappy that I could not suggest an instant solution.

This young man had work-related delayed sleep-wake phase disorder (DSWPD). Recent research from Australia has confirmed the power of bright light therapy to adjust the sleep timing in adolescents and young adults who have this problem.[1] Unfortunately, the body's ability to adapt quickly to changing time zones or sleep schedules is limited by factors we cannot control completely. Normally, at dusk, the suprachiasmatic nucleus (our master clock, located in the hypothalamus) starts to turn off its secretion of hypocretin (also called orexin), and in that way, frees the pineal gland to begin releasing melatonin. While melatonin does not directly cause sleep, it plays an important role in setting our internal clocks. It supports the neurological changes required for sleep to begin.[2] Usually, as we remain awake during the day, our adenosine levels rise, and that brings additional pressure for sleep.

If we make the mistake of flooding our brain with caffeine too late in the day, the brain receptors for that same adenosine can be blocked so thoroughly that the adenosine sleep signal is ineffective. During a ten-year period of very busy medical practice during which I (foolishly) rarely allowed enough time for sleep, even multiple cups of late-in-the-day coffee had no such effect on me. It was only as I learned more about sleep that I realized that I had no unique super-power of caffeine resistance, but rather, that effect was a temporary result of my chronic and profound sleep debt. Now that the chronic sleep deprivation is behind me, I find that even one cup of decaffeinated coffee taken after mid-day can have the normal and expected effect: either temporary trouble falling asleep or middle-of-the-night insomnia.

When we try to change the settings of our body clocks, we are unconsciously asking our body to make adjustments at the biochemical level in order to create a shift in our personal sleep-wake cycle. That's the way it works, whether we change time zones or change shift-work schedules. Cellular biochemistry controls how fast we can make the adjustment. As we've noted, when traveling west, we can adjust (to an earlier setting of our body clocks) by about one hour a day, although using alcohol in flight slows down our adjustment to the new time zone. As we get older, our circadian clocks and the timing of our pineal gland's secretion of melatonin become less reliable, and so does our ability to keep a steady sleep schedule. Our sleep also tends to become more fragmented and less efficient —meaning that we are actually asleep for a smaller fraction of our time in bed when we intend to sleep. That loss of sleep efficiency is not good: it is proportional to lower energy, feelings of depression, loss of memory, and other cognitive functions, as well as to mortality.[3]

The chemical changes that bring about the ticking of our internal clocks have been studied in detail.[4] These changes depend on signals of light and darkness from the environment to adjust the genetically influenced production of special signaling molecules. These are found in the nucleus of every cell throughout our entire body. When these signaling molecules drift out of the cell nucleus into the surrounding cell soup (cytoplasm), they interact with each other to form large molecular assemblies (macromolecules). These assemblies gradually drift back into the cell nucleus, and once there, they block further production of the basic signaling molecules. The re-entry into the nucleus completes the negative feedback loop and allows wake to turn into sleep. Overall, the amount of time it takes to complete these steps of the biochemical cycle is what determines the length of our circadian day. For most of us, that's about 24.2 hours. To keep us functioning on the Earth's 24.0-hour day, we are helped by several zeitgebers—external cues to signal waking and sleeping. These time-givers include daylight (especially short wave-length blue light), mealtimes, work schedules, social interactions, and exercise. Each of us has our own internal clocks, and the length of our natural day is slightly different from other people's. This variability was first recognized in the University of Chicago cave experiment mentioned earlier.

These differences show up, for example, between the roughly 30 percent of us who are genetically programmed to be "night owls" and the minority 4 percent of us who are genetically programmed to be more like "larks." Recent advances in basic science have clarified many details of the interplay between our clock-regulating genes and the chemical changes seen in each of our body's cells that set the length of our own personal "day."[5]

The main points of this chapter are that our bodies have biological clocks in every organ and in every cell, that these determine our personal sleep rhythms, and that our ability to force changes on them is limited by chemical processes we can't control. If we put our sleep-wake cycle out of phase with our internal rhythms, poor health results. If you are experiencing trouble adjusting your sleep schedule to other demands in your life, a sleep specialist can help you make the most effective adjustments available in your particular circumstances.

A DEEPER DIVE FOR THE INTERESTED READER:

While awake, we make several clock-related macromolecules within every cell that has a nucleus. These tiny giants have been given abbreviated names such as Bmal1, PER3, and Clock. They help us regulate our internal clocks through a series of steps and the time it takes to complete the entire sequence. Mutations in the genes that control the production of these molecules determine how long it takes for our personal master clock (in the hypothalamus) to complete one circadian day. For most of us, of course, that's roughly twenty-four hours. As we saw earlier, though, that duration can vary among us.

These macromolecules migrate out of the nucleus into the surrounding cytoplasm, where they collide with other similar macromolecules to form still larger molecular assemblies. Once sufficiently mature, these assemblies migrate back into the cell nucleus, where their size increases still further by combination with additional Clock and Bmal1 molecules. Electron photomicrographs published in 2017 showed the actual growth in their size within the nucleus.[6]

During sleep, the growth in the number of these intranuclear macromolecules begins to inhibit further production of Bmal1 in a negative feedback loop. The pressure for sleep falls with the concentration of Bmal1, and we return to the awake state.

The genes responsible for the production of these macromolecules are subject to mutations like all genes, and such mutations can have significant effects on sleep patterns.

Altered sleep patterns are found in people with mutations of the Clock gene, for example.[7] One such mutation leads to abnormal amounts of non-REM sleep per twenty-four hours. Variations of the PER3 gene are seen in people with atypical amounts of slow-wave sleep during recovery from sleep deprivation.[8]

Scientists now have also shown why we feel so awful when our internal clocks get out of alignment with the clock on our table. Simply changing the time we eat puts the meal out of coordination with our internal clocks and causes striking deviations from the normal hour-by-hour pattern of protein levels found in our bloodstream.[9] When the timing of our sleep is out of phase with our internal rhythms, there are changes in the daily fluctuations of *hundreds* of the RNA molecules that are normally in our blood after being copied from the DNA templates within the nucleus of every cell. Among the molecules whose daily rhythm is upset when sleep is out of phase with our surroundings are Bmal1 and PER3—the very molecules that are most closely involved with the workings of our internal clocks. In other words, sleep patterns that are out of phase with our external environment actually cause molecular-level changes in our internal clock mechanisms.

Although sleep has long been thought to be "of the brain, by the brain, and for the brain,"[10] evidence is piling up that this is an oversimplification and may even have confused the cart with the horse. For example, during sleep-like behavior in the very simple roundworm C. elegans, very little of its "brain" is still active. Just 4 of 150 "brain" cells continue firing during its sleep period.[11] In contrast, the human brain shows even more metabolic activity in sleep (at least during stage REM) than when awake.

The important links between timing of food intake and

human disease show that sleep plays important roles that are not all in the brain. Lopez-Minguez and associates showed that eating within one hour of usual bedtime can reduce tolerance for glucose, compared with eating four hours before usual bedtime.[12] The long-term effect of late eating was shown in a one-month study of more than one hundred college students by McHill and colleagues.[13] They found increased body mass index (BMI) and increased body fat. Food timing also affects the success of intentional weight loss. A study of more than four hundred patients trying to lose weight over a five-month period showed that those who ate "late" lunch lost five pounds less than their "early" lunch peers, even though the "late" lunch group also skipped breakfast more often.[14]

A very irritable forty-three-year-old man reported feeling dangerously sleepy almost all the time for the previous twenty years. His job paid very well, so he was reluctant to quit, but the job required big changes in his work schedule more often than once a week. He felt that he never got enough rest because of the frequent changes in his timing for sleep. In addition to the challenge of the changing eight-hour work shifts, he also had to drive two hours each way between home and the work site. At work, he drove multi-ton ore trucks, and he was constantly afraid he might both die and kill others by falling asleep behind the wheel. His wife was very supportive but noticed he was becoming increasingly short-tempered. She agreed he seemed sleepy most of the time he was home and was very worried that he might have an accident. An overnight sleep study showed no abnormality except for signs of severe sleep deprivation. He did not want a physician's letter to be sent to his employer or the state public health authorities for fear he'd lose his job.

The pressures of industrial activity sometimes lead to work

demands that are simply inconsistent with the limitations imposed by human biology. This has been recognized by the long-haul trucking industry, whose drivers must have certificates stating that they do not have untreated obstructive sleep apnea (OSA, to which many are especially susceptible because of obesity). At least in theory, long-haul truckers are also limited in the number of hours they can drive without a break for sleep. Other industries that employ drivers may not face the same degree of regulation. They may have no legal limits on how often they can be asked for changes in work (and thus sleep) schedules. In states where the tax base depends heavily on affected industries, it may be especially hard for state directors of public health to impose or enforce regulations regarding work hours and schedules. Besides that problem, uninformed supervisors in some industries make shift-change demands on their employees that are certain to cause deterioration of health and at-work alertness of their own workers. One of my patients recently reported being forced to work until midnight one day and yet report to work at 6 a.m. the next. The supervisor probably had no idea how harmful that request was. Shift workers overall report more sick days than workers on more regular schedules. Women seem to have a harder time adjusting to shift work than men and may develop abnormal menstrual cycles.[15]

5

Sleep, Memory, and Learning

As we all look forward to longer lives than we expected when we were very young, we can anticipate a need for continued learning into our advanced years. Gratton and Scott point out that longer careers will become more common, and with those longer careers will come the need for many or even most of us to reinvent ourselves to match the needs of new types of work.[1] We may even need to do this several times in our extended lifetime. As sleep plays a major role in our ability to learn, it seems likely that we'll want to maintain our ability to learn long past our years of formal schooling. This is true especially for our children and younger neighbors because it is they who will likely live even longer than most everyone reading this book.

Each stage of sleep plays a role in memorizing just-learned information, filing it away, and sorting it into quick-access storage or into slower-access long-term storage. The ability to learn new material (whether factual, emotion-related, or part of athletic coordination) depends on sleep coming both before and after the new learning within definite and limited time periods. In this way, both IQ and athletic performance are closely tied to sleep.

In the last few decades, basic scientists around the world have produced powerful new tools that allow sleep scientists and neuroscientists to watch what happens during sleep inside even the deepest parts of our brains. With these new tools they can see how those events influence our memory and recall, and even our very ability to learn. To help the non-expert (including me) follow and understand the importance of recent scientific discoveries, we'll need to take a brief side journey into the science of learning and memory. Those hungry for greater detail will need to look elsewhere, as this is primarily a book about sleep.

Every single day, a huge amount of new information pours into our brains from the experience of all of our senses. Estimates go as high as 11 million bits per second, equaling 950 gigabits (billion bits) sent each day to the thalamus, the brain's inbox.[2] How the brain distributes this new information varies depending on the type of information. For ease of understanding, we'll ignore most of those differences here. In any case, the brain can't handle the new information as fast as the deluge comes in. That leads us to the conclusion that a large amount of "data compression" must somehow take place in the brain. For a new memory to be stored, it may need to pass through conscious awareness, and that's the bottleneck for processing new information. Robert Lucky of Bell Labs has estimated that the bandwidth of the conscious mind is limited to processing roughly 50 to 120 bits of information per second. That would correspond to a daily total of less than ten gigabits, but that is just over 1 percent of the information flood that we need to process every day. Small errors in these estimates wouldn't really change the main conclusion: the only way we can handle our daily load of new information is by using data compression. On the other hand, you will probably be very happy to learn that we humans can process information faster than a mouse.[3]

We collect information sent by our senses (mainly sight, smell, taste, touch, position, and hearing). But we also collect information with more editorial content: something is beautiful, foul smelling, hostile, or friendly, for example. This mighty stream of data enters the brain for temporary storage through the hippocampus, located in the best-protected part of the brain on both the right and left sides. Information processing then determines whether a particular bit of information will be kept on file or can safely be forgotten (or, more likely, placed in the brain's deep-freeze storage in the basement). That selection step appears to be mainly the responsibility of the thalamus, located very near and just above the hippocampus. Memories to be filed are sent "upstairs" to the cerebral cortex, that is, directly to the outermost and most modern layers of the brain. Information that seems important enough for immediate retrieval ("Where's the brake pedal on this new rental car?") is then re-filed in nearby clusters of brain cells just below the outer cortex.

Using functional MRI, investigators have shown (not surprisingly) that we humans differ a lot from each other in the way our brains work. This little fact was intuited decades ago by the late and brilliant Cal Tech physicist Richard Feynman.[4] At the same time, these studies have also shown surprising similarities from one person to another in the way our brains handle memories of similar topics and how we recall them later. Fascinating recent developments in this field have been very clearly described by Shen.[5] Scientists observed which parts of the brain light up when volunteers are exposed to new information and which parts light up when they are shown pictures they have seen before. That way, the investigators could see in real time where a new memory was stored and from where it was later retrieved. Of special interest to us, sleep is the time when much or even most of the after-the-fact or "offline" processing of new memories occurs.

That processing is essential for later recall. Since the processing of new memories occurs mainly during sleep, this makes sleep absolutely crucial for any learning. These studies also offer a clue into how the sleeping brain can discover associations among memories that the awake brain has not recognized. These discoveries happen especially during stage REM, when both current and older memories may be simultaneously activated due to some common feature (such as emotion, smell, sound, or pattern). By allowing disparate (new and old) memories to be simultaneously activated and thus linked, newly recognized associations may be a—or maybe even *the*—primary basis of creativity. Why is this all important to us? The upshot is that different steps in the normal handling of new information (i.e., learning) require different parts of the symphony of sleep to be available to the learner—and each part of the symphony must be available within specific windows of time before or after exposure to the new information (such as in class). Therefore, if you want to be a good student—whether of welding or atomic physics—you would be wise to keep to a rather stable sleep-wake schedule. That will maximize your effectiveness at gaining new knowledge.

As we'll discuss further in chapter 10, it is the deeper stages of sleep that are especially important to processing and retaining new knowledge. We can see this in people whose sleep patterns cause loss of time in deep sleep. For example, between ages six through twelve, the percent of sleep time spent in stage 1 (shallow sleep) is inversely proportional to IQ and learning ability: the more stage 1, the lower the learning ability. The same is true of patients with OSA: the more severe it is, the less the ability to learn. While the latter will be discussed further in chapter 10, what both of these measures imply is that it's the deeper sleep stages that are important in processing new information and in the brain's ability to manipulate stored information.

Information processing by our brain requires several parts of the brain to be involved in an orderly sequence. Exact details vary with the type of information being handled. For example, in stage 2 sleep, sleep spindles are sometimes the electrical clue that information is being passed back and forth between the thalamus and the cerebral cortex. Not surprisingly, the amount of spindle activity is proportional to the consolidation of new memory (i.e., sorting and filing for long-term storage). Sleep spindles seen during stage 2 also represent cortical-to-subcortical information transfer from processing centers to rapid access storage. As we might expect, that activity is increased during sleep that follows new learning, including learning of new motor skills. This discovery not only supports the importance of sleep for athletes in training, but it hints that measures of sleep spindles are also a reflection of general IQ. These discoveries underline the importance of adequate sleep to students of all ages and in every field of study.

Slow-wave or delta sleep (seen in stages 3 and 4) also supports the consolidation of some new memories (especially those providing context and color). New contextual learning is stronger after a "class" if during a post-class ninety-minute nap there are lots of spindles seen in slow-wave sleep—just as we noted for motor memory during stage 2 sleep. Retention of new smell-associated memory is better if the odor is presented again during later slow-wave sleep, but not if the odor is re-presented during wake or stage REM.[6] Functional MRI images during slow-wave sleep in these studies show lighting up of the same hippocampal neurons with odor re-exposure during slow-wave sleep as during the original odor exposure during wakefulness. Slow-wave sleep is also needed for the extinction of less important memories.

In stage REM, the number of eye movements per minute after a learning session (class) is proportional to the learning ability of the subject.[7] During REM and slow-wave sleep, the very fast "ripple" waves detected at the hippocampus are seen during memory replay and consolidation activity.[8] Ripple waves are detected only during research studies—they are too fast to be recorded during routine clinical sleep studies (overnight polysomnograms). They can reveal individual nerve cells firing at rates up to eight hundred or even one thousand times per second.

The strength of new, emotionally negative memory is increased during REM sleep and is also increased when theta waves (four to seven waves per second) are detected on the scalp over the brain's prefrontal cortex. If a recent memory of sound is reactivated by exposure to the same sound during REM sleep, the electrical activity of the cortex increases. This means that the recent memory of that sound has already been incorporated into the brain cells of the cortex. This may be part of the mechanism for causing PTSD among combat veterans.

The main take-home message of this chapter is not so much the technical details of where and how the brain works during sleep to form our memories but rather to show that learning is very much dependent on adequate amounts and particular stages of sleep. There is simply overwhelming published scientific evidence that enough hours—and appropriate timing—of sleep have very large effects on our ability to learn. This is true of sleep before study and also after study. It is true for factual learning and for physical skills learning. It is true for contextual learning. It is true for infants, children, and adults. If you are trying to learn anything at all—a new language, a new musical instrument, a new sport, or even (maybe especially) the basic education for your life—you simply cannot avoid the importance of getting adequate sleep. An excellent in-depth review of related studies is available for the curious reader in the book *Why We Sleep*.[9]

6

Sleep and Dreams

Whether the Old Testament was written by man or not, in either case, it shows that even long ago, there was some understanding of the amazing power of dreams. By that I mean showing truths not recognized before the dreamer fell asleep. In the book of Genesis chapter 20, King Abimelech has taken from Abraham the beautiful woman Sarah. Abraham has described Sarah to the king as his (Abraham's) own sister, but in reality, she was both his wife and also his half-sister. Abraham told this half-truth to avoid being murdered by the jealous King Abimelech. Now asleep but waking suddenly from a dream, Abimelech recognizes the truth: he has just barely avoided the sin of sleeping with another man's wife.[1] We will return to this mysterious power of dreams later in this chapter —when we explore how dreams can help us understand earlier events better than we did at the time we were in the process of living those events.

The same theme appears in the nineteenth-century *Remembrances of Things Past* by Marcel Proust.[2] The main character dreams of his childhood, remembering a moment when, with a group of adults, he was watching lantern slides projected on a wall. In his dream many years later, he suddenly recognizes relationships that existed among the adults with him at that earlier time but were completely unrecognized by him then. As he reflects in his dream on that scene, he suddenly understands what had been hidden from him for many years since that scene.

Yet a third feature attributed to dreams is part of the biblical story of Joseph. While imprisoned in Egypt, Joseph is allowed to interpret a mysterious and frightening dream experienced by the pharaoh. He tells the pharaoh that the mysterious dream is foretelling a seven-year drought and famine that will devastate Egypt after seven years of abundant crops. In a kingdom totally dependent for food on the annual floods of the Nile River, prolonged drought is terrifying news. Fortunately, Joseph's interpretation of the dream gives him time to plan and prepare ways to help Pharoah save his people from starvation.[3]

So, how do dreams arise? Dreams occur only when collections of neurons in the brain (circuits) are turned on (activated), and that happens without stimulation from outside the body (self-activation). The electrical signals indicating the start of a dream come from the reticular activating system in the brain stem—a very primitive part of the brain. (By primitive, I mean that similar structures are found even in very primitive creatures that have been present on this earth far longer than man.) Perhaps that indicates that dreams are an essential feature of our lives. In any case, the order of activation of various circuits is unpredictable—seemingly random. Not only is the input gate to our brain (for new information from the environment, the thalamus) temporarily closed during dreaming, but so is the output gate, which might otherwise result in dangerous muscle activity during violent dreams.

In contrast to the gradual onset of sleep due to the normal transition from a brain bathed in alerting neurotransmitters (such as norepinephrine and serotonin) to one bathed in a sedating neurotransmitter (acetylcholine), sleep can be produced immediately by injection of acetylcholine directly into the medial part of the pons (in the midbrain). As a result of the changed chemical milieu of the brain cells when dreaming begins, most of us lose the ability to pay attention to our surroundings and the ability to have reflective thoughts.

As the high-speed signals of nerve-cell traffic pass back and forth between regions of the brain, older memories are brought back online, where they can interact with new memories of the day. The resulting blended memories are evident in complex dreams that mix current affairs with old events and may well be the neural basis of what is called creativity. (See chapter 8.)

When circuits are activated during stage REM in the multi-media cortex part of our brain (deep to the ears), the result is that we become aware of images, sound, color, and motion. When other circuits are activated, our ability to be skeptical and pass judgment is suppressed. Our brain's higher centers somehow create a narrative to place these varying multi-media images into some kind of coherent story (narrative). The fact that the narrative often makes no rational sense causes no distress to the dreamer because his/her ability to pass judgment is temporarily suppressed. Modern medical technology, including functional MRI (imaging), allows scientists to know when metabolic activity in any part of the brain is either suppressed or increased. As the role of a number of brain centers is known in terms of thought and mental abilities, such studies reinforce the evidence collected from electrical signal (electroencephalogram) studies. As sleep stages vary within each part of the symphony of sleep, chemical influences on neuronal excitability shift and modulate dreams.

By waking people from sleep, scientists have learned that adults dream during about 25 percent of their total sleep time. Dreaming seems to occupy a larger fraction of REM sleep as we get older. Cartwright found that three- to four-year-olds reported dreaming only 27 percent of the time when they were awakened from REM.[4] By ages five to seven, Cartwright's subjects reported dreams in 31 percent of the REM awakenings, but by ages eleven to thirteen, the number had risen to 66 percent. In adulthood, it was 85 percent. Those differing numbers are consistent with the idea that a major role for stage REM in uterine life and early childhood is to support the creation of the many neural networks essential to meeting life's demands, while REM dreams of later life may serve different purposes.

In addition to the 25 percent of our average night that includes dreaming (especially REM), there is another 25 percent of the night that has mental activity that we can unearth by awakening and questioning the sleeper. In contrast, people awakened from slow-wave or delta sleep (adding up to 20 percent or less of our nights) are unable to describe anything that was happening in their brain. Even though there is clear electrical brain-wave activity, they have no dreams or thoughts to report. We don't know whether that means there are no thoughts during that time or rather that the thoughts are not accessible to the awake brain. The brain is clearly processing information, but that is somehow happening below the level of conscious awareness. Perhaps the mental activity of delta sleep corresponds to the views of Freud and Jung regarding the activity of the unconscious and subconscious mind, to be discussed later in this chapter.

Although dreaming occurs in other stages of sleep, it is especially prominent in stage REM. The dreams of REM are different in several ways from dreams of other sleep stages. Most importantly, REM dreams have significant emotional content. That is seen even in the youngest newborn infants, whose facial grimaces and smiles are generally thought to reflect emotions. It is possible that the process of being born creates emotion-laden memories, but it is doubted by many that newborns have any other significant emotional baggage they need to process through dreaming. Some argue that dream content itself may even have little or no significance. In any case, dream specialists from the field of emotional health hold widely differing views about the significance of dream content.

Another typical feature of REM dreams is that they always have a role for the self—that is, the person having the dream. They are colorful, active, and often geographically inconsistent. They are unreal, and none of these unrealistic features arouses any doubt or suspicion in the mind of the dreamer during those dreams. During the dream, there is simply no awareness that the action taking place in the dream is not true to life. There's not any concern about the abruptly shifting cast of characters or the sudden changes of time or location of the dream's action. These mental gymnastics have features of psychosis, such as the presence of unreality, the absence of disbelief, and the lack of awareness of the dreamer's external environment. And yet, despite all that psychotic-like mental activity during the dream, the dreamer again awakens within minutes or hours and again has normal mental function. Let's count that as yet another amazing power of our brains during sleep.

In contrast, dreams of non-REM sleep are largely without

color; with some exceptions, they're emotionally blander, and they're less complicated. They seem more or less like realistic reporting of actual personal history—especially of the day just past. They usually have a somewhat negative emotional tone. For example, night terrors are dreams that arise from delta (slow-wave) sleep. Their content may be pure emotion with little action or cast of characters. The child in the midst of such a dream is largely unaware of his surroundings and can't be comforted or awakened even by his parents until the terrifying dream fades by itself. The next morning, he remembers nothing about it except possibly the frightening emotional content. As delta sleep occurs especially in the early part of the night, that's when night terrors occur.

Adding to the evidence that dreaming happens at the same time as activation of certain parts of the brain is yet another discovery—this one with regard to seizures. Temporal lobe seizures (corresponding to uncontrolled activation in the temporal lobes of the brain) are associated with dreams, and if that part of the brain (parietal multi-modular cortex) is injured or damaged by disease, dreaming can no longer occur.

Similarly, if the deep frontal white matter (cortex) is damaged, the ability to dream is also lost. So even though dreams originate with activation of the brain stem, loss of either of the above parts of the brain makes dreaming impossible even with direct electrical stimulation of the brain stem.

Let's look at how memories of dream content are studied and what limitations those methods bring. Some spontaneously remembered dreams have been dictated or written down directly by the dreamer or by a therapist or scientist later, after questioning. Most investigations, though, have depended on dreams reported just as the dreamer has been awakened, purposely to ask what was being dreamed at that moment. That might mean that the record is of the final dream of the night or that the remainder of the night may now have been affected by the artificial awakenings. Some subjects recall only rare or even no dreams under these conditions, while others recall dreams very consistently. Those who have limited dream recall do not seem to be physically or mentally unhealthy despite that lack of dreaming—or at least the lack of dream reports. Some investigators believe that information means that dream content—or at least the ability to recall dream content—is of no biological importance.

In the case of REM dreams, if arousal from REM does not occur within ninety seconds of the dream, the dream can never be recalled. After ninety seconds, the dream will be lost forever unless it has already entered memory. That is true because dreams can only be recorded by the brain in the presence of norepinephrine. (Norepinephrine is one of the most important neurotransmitters of the awake brain, along with serotonin.) During REM, the secretion of both norepinephrine and serotonin is turned off and rapidly disappears from the environment of the brain's neurons.

When spontaneous activation of brain circuits begins in sleep, the resulting dream images relate to actual events of the day, but soon, other brain circuits are also activated. These may relate to older experiences somehow connected to this day's experiences. Emotional content is the strongest link to older memories: the new and the old sharing the same emotion. The images brought back from storage may have little in common with new images of the day except for their emotional content. The mind's attempt to tie these separate strands of memory together into some understandable dream narrative—especially in REM—is thought to be what produces the typically bizarre character of REM dreams.

Although the search to understand the nature of dreams and their meaning in our lives is probably as old as man's ability to think abstract thoughts, the tools needed to improve our understanding are not much older than the length of a long human life. Even so, for millennia mystics, shamans, and therapists have offered to provide special insights into the significance of dream content. This tradition flows from the Book of Genesis and the Delphic Oracle in pre-Christian Greece on through time to the city of Vienna at the end of the nineteenth century and to now-contemporary psychiatry and clinical psychology.

In Vienna, at the end of the nineteenth century, Sigmund Freud studied and wrote beautifully to show others how the content of human dreams was related to unconscious desires and to conflicts within the minds of his patients.[5] He called dreams "the royal road to the unconscious" and felt that the role of the psychoanalyst was to help the patient discover the emotional conflicts hiding in his unconscious and causing his turmoil. He had no way to prove his conclusions except the successful outcomes reported in his case histories. He was nonetheless able to generate very wide acceptance and widespread use of dream interpretation for the treatment of mental illness. Some academic psychiatrists have tended to regard his work as never scientifically validated, [6] and as a result, psychoanalysis was simply not taught in the medical school I attended. Freud described neurotic conflicts as lying somewhere in the brain below thc level of consciousness (except during dreams) yet still being able to have powerful effects on the behavior of people during their waking hours. Despite strong opposing opinions among some sleep scientists, later in this chapter, we will review some evidence that supports his view: that emotions we're not consciously aware of can indeed influence our behavior.

Another major effort to understand and use dreams in psychotherapy was led by Carl Jung. He believed that the narrative of dreams was best understood in terms of symbolism: that the dreams reflected hidden emotional conflicts symbolized by the dream narratives of the patient. He urged therapists to look beyond sexual conflicts to the larger life histories of their patients for better insight into the causes of their distress. He also stressed that many hidden conflicts stemmed from patients having lost touch with their most important primitive emotions, such as fear and aggressiveness.

In parallel with these observations about the hallucinatory features of REM dreams, there are now synchronized neuroimaging findings. Dreaming is accompanied by decreased metabolic activity at the brain's main center of judgment and reflective thought (the upper lateral part of the brain cortex at the front of our head). At the same time, studies show increased metabolic activity at the location hosting multimodular image creation (parietal brain cortex on the sides of the head). Also, at the same time, there's activity of nerve cells in the limbic system and the basal forebrain, which are the main centers of emotion and instinctive behaviors. I suspect that Freud would have been thrilled to learn that the "I" (that is, the sense of self) has now been localized to the prefrontal cortex at the sides of the front of the head. It is metabolically and electrically quiet during dream-consciousness. During some dreams, the hippocampus—where recent memory is located—is also quiet, and at the same time, factual (declarative) memory is also impaired.

Dream occurrence and dream content are governed by the emotional relevance of the dream's subject matter and by the active association of recent memories with older ones. These are supported by changes in the chemical environment of the brain's one hundred billion neurons.

Dream reports that are obtained by waking volunteers from non-REM sleep are thought to represent the unconscious (Freud's term). Contemporary sleep specialists might call it the subconscious. The brain is processing information without our being at all aware of that activity. When rats are studied during sleep soon after they have been learning their way around a new maze, the same brain circuits that were active during the learning time in the maze are again activated during non-REM sleep. In human volunteers with brain electrodes placed to study their epileptic seizures, the same cells active during daytime learning are again spontaneously reactivated during sleep and are also active during dreams recalling that earlier learning activity.

It is the changing chemical environment of brain cells that brings about the change from being awake to being asleep. Secretion of glutamate or other neurotransmitters within synapses (the connections between nerve cells) makes each neuron more or less excitable by adjusting a characteristic feature of all cells called trans-membrane electric potential (the difference in voltage measured between the outside of the cell and the fluid contained within its cell membrane).

Within any synapse, increased secretion of glutamate brings greater excitability of the neurons. Secretion of GABA (gamma-aminobutyric acid, another neurotransmitter) within synapses has exactly the opposite effect. Instead of the overwhelming influence of norepinephrine and serotonin in the brain that's present when we're awake, it is the increasing influence of acetylcholine that causes the gradual onset of sleep. The rising tide of acetylcholine causes decreased alertness, effectively putting the mind offline from the rest of the brain, and we are asleep. In contrast to the slow and steady change in brain state brought about by these chemical influences over a number of minutes, the electrical activation of neural circuits takes place within milliseconds (thousands of a second), and the related dream imagery also changes very quickly. Neuromodulation (adjustment of neuronal activity) by changes in the brain's chemical environment occurs within all phases of sleep. In non-REM sleep, the brain's waking secretion of norepinephrine and serotonin is cut down by half. In stage REM, that secretion stops entirely, as already noted.

Is there value in helping someone understand the emotional or psychological basis of his or her dreams? While that remains unproven using the formal methods of scientific investigation, what is beyond doubt is that dreaming of emotional conflicts is associated with recovery from emotional distress and from some psychopathologies. Moderately depressed people often dream about the subject of their depression (after divorce, for example). They all tend to be less depressed after a night with related dreams. The ones who maintain the improved mood through the next day are more likely to recover from their depression within the next few months than those whose mood sours again by the end of the next day. What a contribution to mental health might be made by showing how to make the improved mood last all day.

It is also known that during depression, slow-wave sleep is decreased. At the same time, REM starts earlier in the night, lasts longer, and has much less dream activity. There is also increased activity of the brain in areas controlling emotion and executive function. Poor quality sleep is typically followed by a return of depression. Learning how to prevent sleep from deteriorating in people with bipolar disorder would also be a huge contribution to mental health. Mood-stabilizing drugs aim to accomplish exactly that.

Evidence like this leads to the conclusion that dreaming plays an important role in taming negative emotions. Not only is that desirable from the point of view of one's own emotional stability and happiness, but it is also an important group and individual survival tactic. This is especially true in societies where a powerful leader bearing a grudge may cause severe or even fatal consequences to another member of his clan. That kind of hostility and danger to others in the clan could weaken the entire clan by decreasing group coherence.

Dreaming has two additional benefits that are important for survival. Dreaming permits memory updates to help combine newly learned information with what was previously known. Dreaming also allows the brain to reorganize in view of new experiences and allows one to update one's personal understanding of the world, including what Cartwright called "updating the software of the self."

One way of looking at the relationships between thinking and dreaming is to consider that there are three types of thinking: conscious thinking, unconscious thinking, and subconscious thinking. Subconscious thinking is present in the background while we dream. The evidence for this comes from reports of mental activity of subjects awakened from non-REM sleep. Unconscious thinking corresponds to the ongoing mental activity (information processing) during slow-wave sleep—but subjects awakened from slow-wave sleep have literally no recall of any mental activity at the time they are awakened. Nevertheless, the brain centers activated during new learning sessions are also activated during slow-wave sleep that follows the learning sessions.

Scientists also infer brain activity during slow-wave sleep

from the disorders called parasomnias (see chapter 11) that arise typically out of slow-wave sleep. It is obvious that at least part of the brain must be active during sleepwalking or the various other "motor parasomnias," but scientists have been unable to retrieve any verbal evidence of that brain activity from their patients. From this, they conclude that different parts of the brain may not be in the same stage of sleep at any particular time. Maybe this can help sleep specialists understand better the problem of sleep state misperception or paradoxical insomnia. In patients with this disorder, a sleep study may clearly show brain wave patterns of sleep, but the patient may insist the next day that he slept little or not at all and that he felt awake throughout the night. (See the vignette regarding my architect patient in chapter 9.) Sometimes, he can even report accurately on events that took place during the night when his brain waves indicated he was asleep. Taken together, the evidence now available suggests that the mind is active throughout the twenty-four-hour day, although some uncertainty remains about whether it is active during normal slow-wave sleep.

One of the problems faced by some veterans returning from war is post-traumatic stress disorder (PTSD). Among its prominent features are recurring and very disturbing nightmares.[7] Sleep scientists have looked hard for objective neurological clues to the diagnosis. Along with the shift in how memories are encoded and processed, which we touched on in chapter 5, there may be clues within the nightmares that characterize the disorder. Recently, Dutch investigators found that characteristic shifts in the brain waves of PTSD sufferers may provide such a clue.[8] They wrote that those who did have the disorder had a decrease in slow-wave electrical brain oscillations during non-REM sleep compared with control subjects who had similar histories of trauma but were not suffering from PTSD. This was especially true over the frontal parts of the brain, and this change in the "power spectrum" was associated with insomnia. Perhaps we can look forward to an application of the rocking bed studies (which brought increased slow-wave sleep)[9] as a treatment for the decrease of slow-wave sleep seen in PTSD patients.

The role of sleep in treatment is not limited to the benefits of dreams. Everyone is familiar with the power of sleep to restore a sense of well-being during (especially viral) illness. Energy improves, ability to concentrate improves, and malaise recedes.

Shakespeare knew it four hundred years ago: "sleep that kniteth up the ravel'd sleeve of care. . . . balm of hurt minds."[10] By automatically shutting off secretion of the alerting neurotransmitter norepinephrine in the brain during stage REM, we are able to replay traumatic memories as dreams, with a lessened degree of anxiety than would otherwise be the case. As dreams of traumatic events occur again and again, there is a gradual lowering of the associated anxiety level. The way this happens may involve the formation of "extinction memories."[11]

Using similar lines of evidence, Cartwright found that recovery from divorce-related depression during the first year after divorce was dependent on dreaming about the divorce. Most patients gradually lost the negative emotional content of their REM dreams, but those who remained depressed had not. In the latter group, waking them during REM dreams brought temporary relief: they felt less depressed after waking for the day.[12] Even though sleep is generally beneficial to health in many ways, the use of sleep deprivation as a treatment for depression has proved to be quickly and at least temporarily effective.[13] The use of sleep in the management of psychiatric patients has been explored more broadly by Harvey and colleagues.[14,15] For immediately effective treatment of severe depression, sleep deprivation is both effective and safe.[16]

In this chapter, we've seen how dreams differ from conscious thought. We've seen that they nonetheless portray the same themes of thought and actual activities of the day just past. We've seen how the dreams of REM allow the memory of new experiences to be mixed with those of long ago, resulting in new insights and even some "aha!" moments. We've seen how dreams can influence daytime emotions and even have effects on mental illness. We've also noted that the absence of sleep (and thus of dreaming) can also be useful in psychiatric treatment.

If your dreams seem unusually troubling, consulting a therapist who specializes in emotional health can usually provide guidance and relief.

7

Sleep and Athletic Performance

If you're an amateur or professional athlete aiming to perform at your best and with safety, you'll want to have enough sleep. This important news is now widely known among coaches, exercise physiologists, and athletes themselves. Both the amount of sleep and the time when sleep occurs are important, but in general, lots of sleep is crucial to athletic success. As we noted earlier, Ariana Huffington reported that tennis great Roger Federer arranged to have ten to twelve hours of sleep on nights before his most important championship matches.[1]

Published scientific studies have confirmed what Roger Federer discovered for himself. The National Collegiate Athletic Association (NCAA), for example, published their sleep recommendations for college athletes in 2019[2]—perhaps unsurprisingly, eight hours per night. The year before that, Knufinke reported on studies in ninety-eight elite karate athletes: he found that longer sleep was associated with faster reaction times.[3] Following a night of partial sleep deprivation, his athletes responded to a half-hour nap in the early afternoon by showing greater alertness and better physical performance. Even after a normal night of sleep, those brief naps still brought improved alertness and cognitive function.[4]

People are known to vary in the timing of their most alert periods (see chapter 4), so Anderson studied the influence of time of day on performance among swimmers. Both the natural circadian rhythm of the individual swimmer (lark versus owl) and the inherited genotype for the gene PER3 affected the time of day when the swimmer would perform best. In other words, who gets the medal may depend on what time of day the competition is held.[5]

Loss of sleep also brings a greater risk of injury during active sports. So does the chance of getting ill in the following week. Fitzgerald studied the training load and amount of sleep of forty-four nationally competitive male Australian football players for a complete season of more than ten months. He found that when sleep time was reduced, there was a greater chance of the athletes getting sick within the next week. Training load, on the other hand, did not affect the risk of illness.[6]

How much athletic performance is affected by sleep deprivation depends on the sport. Kirschen reviewed nineteen studies of sleep and performance across twelve different sports.[7] He concluded that sports requiring speed, tactical strategy, and technical skill were the ones most affected by variations in sleep. Brief changes in sleep had less effect on athletic performance than longer-term changes, as we might have expected. A separate (and massive) study of almost one hundred twenty thousand Chinese children ages nine to fifteen gave similar results. Both average speed during a fifty-meter dash and results of long-distance endurance runs were best in children with more than nine hours of sleep each night. They were worst in children with fewer than seven hours each night.[8]

Even an afternoon nap of twenty minutes helps athletes recover from the effects of too little sleep the night before. After a "rescue nap," runners ran longer before exhaustion and also had a decreased sense of effort during their run.[9] Ultramarathon runners seem to know this intuitively. Taking naps and extending nighttime sleep hours were the two strategies employed most often among 636 such athletes preparing for their ultramarathon runs of 36-60 hours or more.[10]

During another study covering twenty-six netball matches, young elite female athletes tested the effect of their nap habits on match days. The girls who took a nap (lasting no longer than twenty minutes) showed increased jump speed and better overall performance as judged by their own coaches.[11]

Readers will probably not be surprised to learn that fitness in older adults varies with time spent in moderate to vigorous physical activity. Constantly wearing accelerometers to measure how vigorously they moved, 122 older Australian men and women spent a week recording how much time they spent asleep, how much time in sedentary activities, and how much time they were physically more active. For every fifteen minutes spent in physical activity, there was a measurable increase in aerobic capacity (a measure of fitness), a decrease in BMI (a stand-in for weight), and a decrease in waist-to-hip ratio (a measure of obesity). For each quarter hour less than the group's average spent in daily physical activity, there were even larger changes in the opposite (less desirable) direction.[12]

Motor memory is also influenced by sleep: speed and accuracy both improve when typing lessons are either followed by sleep or preceded by sleep.[13] Brain MRI studies show that just-learned motor skills are stored in long-term subcortical (subconscious) memory banks, especially in the part of the brain called the motor cortex. The gains in skill are in proportion to the amount of stage 2 sleep during the first night following training, especially during the last few hours of that night's sleep. It's interesting to speculate whether that sub-cortical storage of motor skills and other memory corresponds to the "thinking fast" described by Nobel laureate Daniel Kahneman in his book *Thinking, Fast and Slow.*[14]

Conversely, short hours of sleep in young athletes are dangerous. Chronic lack of sleep increases the risk of sports injuries in adolescent athletes. Child athletes getting nine hours of sleep per night had a less than 20 percent risk of injury, while those averaging only six hours per night had a risk greater than 70 percent. With average sleep hours in between those two extremes, the risks of injury were also in between the two extremes.[15]

Overall, it's hard to escape the conclusion that adequate hours of sleep are important to athletic success and safety. So if you want to improve your level of playing ____ (fill in the blank), aim to get more sleep.

8

Sleep and the "Aha!" Moment

Humans sleep less than other primates (eight hours per night in humans, compared with ten or even fifteen hours per night in other primates). On the other hand, we humans typically have much more stage REM (20 to 25 percent) compared with only about 9 percent among other primates. Could that richness of REM in our sleep have anything to do with what seems like far greater complexity of human societies compared with other primate societies? There are two aspects of stage REM that might help explain that mystery. For one thing, during stage REM, we experience seemingly random associations of what look like completely unrelated memories. This allows new information to be connected with stored older memories, leading to new insights —in other words, to creativity and moments of clarity.

This effect of sleep on creative thinking was first shown to me by the teacher of a Carleton College math class (on simultaneous differential equations). He (Kenneth O. May) suggested that if I just couldn't find the answer to a tough problem, I should try sleeping on it—and it worked! After a night's sleep, the answer to a particular mind-bender of a problem (for me) popped into my mind as soon as I looked at the problem again the next day. A far more important example of this sleep-fosters-creativity phenomenon was demonstrated about 150 years ago when the great Russian chemist Dmitri Mendeleev awoke from a deep sleep. He was familiar with many properties of all the chemical elements known at that time, but for ten years he had tried unsuccessfully to determine how they were related to each other. Awakening from a dream about that problem with a start, he went to his desk and immediately wrote out the chart demonstrating how the elements were related to each other. Since that day, every high school student of chemistry has become familiar with Mendeleev's Periodic Table of the Elements.

There's some evidence that maximum creativity requires both adequate stage REM and also REM dreams that are related to the problem waiting to be solved. Even naps are capable of supporting this kind of creativity if dreams related to the problem show up during the naps. Not only is retention of new factual memory supported by stage REM, but understanding is also improved. Subjects were shown apparently unrelated numbers and then allowed to sleep. After that, they were asked to find the "rule" relating the numbers to each other. Among those whose sleep included REM, the success rate was three times as great as among those whose sleep had not included REM. Another big surprise from that study was that success in discovering the hidden rule required some REM, but was not proportional to the amount of REM. It was instead proportional to the amount of slow-wave sleep.[1] Further studies showed that success was also related to the number of times the brain switched sleep stages each night between non-REM and REM. That finding meant that both

REM and non-REM sleep were needed for the brain to process the remembered information (numbers) and find the hidden rule. It's also important that even before sleep started, the brain had already stored all the information it needed to solve the problem, but the creative act of solution-finding required manipulation of that information—and that could only happen by interactions between REM and slow-wave sleep.[2] Isn't it amazing how much is happening in our brains while we're quietly asleep?

The second way that REM may have played a big role in the development of human societies is in helping us defuse explosively unpleasant memories. Research from Harvard has shown that the themes of REM dreams do correspond roughly to the themes of thoughts recorded in daytime personal diaries, especially in terms of their emotional content.[3] In that way, REM dreams allow review of troubling experiences and so lead to a progressively calmer emotional response to the original upsetting event. So, repetition of the dream safely allows gradual extinction of the unpleasantness associated with the memories. This emotional recalibration occurs through renewed activity in the right and left prefrontal cortex part of the brain—and that is the seat of rational thought and judgment. At the same time, there is decreased activity in the amygdala and cingulate cortex, which are the centers of emotional responses. By gradually reducing the emotional response to an unpleasant memory, this recalibration permits future interactions within the society to be less hostile. This might be especially important in the case of a powerful male leader (think gorillas) following an unpleasant experience with another individual member of his troop. In that way, reduced conflict within the societal group would promote group stability—thanks in part to stage REM (and to dreams, as we reviewed in chapter 6).

In people suffering from PTSD, some so-far unknown factor has interfered with the normal extinction of an unpleasant memory of one or more traumatic events.[4] Convincing evidence suggests that this effect is due at least in part to the release of stress hormones such as norepinephrine during stressful dreams. As a result, treatment of PTSD with Prazosin (a blocker of catecholamine hormones like norepinephrine) has met with some success. It seems probable, though, that PTSD is a complex disorder, since not all PTSD patients respond to treatment with Prazosin.

Studies have shown that about 20 percent of people can actually control some aspects of their dreams. Volunteers were told to remember one group of words shown to them before sleep and were told not to remember a different group shown in the same session. They were able to direct their brains to remember the target group better than the other group. This phenomenon is considered part of what has been called lucid dreaming. Lucid dreamers are also able during sleep to give signals with their eyes and to control breathing movements by controlling dream content.[5] Lucid dreaming also allows some people to control the direction of dreams. For example, I'm sometimes able to make my dream return to a thread involving something I don't want to lose after the dream changes directions. The desired thread is sometimes (but not always) erotic. Whether it is possible to use this ability to encourage creative solutions to troublesome problems is not clear, but there is some evidence of a link between creativity and the hallucinations of narcolepsy type 1.[6] When you're facing a problem you can't quite solve, you may want to follow the advice of my distinguished math professor and sleep on it!

9

Why Can't I Sleep?

A woman in her seventies complained that for more than twenty-five years she'd had trouble falling asleep. She had used sleeping pills every night for nearly twenty years and couldn't stop. She felt socially isolated because she was afraid to attend public events or even to entertain at her own home any longer: either she might embarrass herself by falling asleep in public or be too stimulated to be able to sleep at all—even with her usual sleeping pill. She was worried that something might have damaged her brain permanently, causing the insomnia. Years earlier she had been very active as a host, and she was now very unhappy with her life.

She asked, "Why can't I sleep?"

At least forty million other Americans ask that question. Nearly all of us can remember at least one time in our life when something very upsetting happened and kept us awake thinking about it—sometimes all night. Think again of Shakespeare's Macbeth wandering sleepless around his castle (after murdering his king): he complains, "Macbeth hath murdered sleep!"[1] It can be far less dramatic thoughts that keep us awake.

Temporary insomnia usually lasts only a few days and resolves by itself. No treatment is needed except possibly reassurance. When trouble falling asleep or staying asleep through the night lasts longer, but still fewer than three months, we call it short-term insomnia. Often, insomnia continues more than a few days because the sufferer has tried to get rid of it with remedies that have the opposite effect.

A successful businesswoman complained of many months of interrupted sleep that was interfering with her otherwise enjoyable work with her business clientele. She couldn't recall what started her pattern of disturbed sleep, but she often fell asleep fairly easily. The problem was that she awoke some hours later and seemed to toss and turn for hours after that. For the past few months she had been taking a night cap of white wine to help her fall asleep, and it had worked. Unfortunately, it had made the middle-of-the-night awakenings much worse. They were now a daily occurrence. After review of her sleep rituals (sleep hygiene), we concluded together that the night-cap was the most likely cause of her worsened sleep-maintenance insomnia.

When alcohol is taken near bedtime, the alcohol in the blood eases the change from wake to sleep. As the liver begins to metabolize the circulating alcohol over the next three to five hours, it has an opposite effect: wakefulness. Once we reviewed this information, she resolved to stop the night-cap habit. This one step often resolves the problem of troublesome sleep maintenance insomnia.

We don't completely understand why women are more subject to chronic insomnia than men. An inherited factor seems likely to play a role,[2] leading to persistent over-activation of the sympathetic nervous system. What results is continued activity during the night of the brain's reticular activating system, which includes the hippocampus, the amygdala and the thalamus. This implies that external stimuli are forwarded into the brain—not normal during sleep—getting processed and then producing emotional responses to these external stimuli. These events can happen only if there's an (abnormally) open condition of the "thalamic gate." It may be that the constant alerting of the brain in response to these inputs inhibits development of stage 2 and deeper delta sleep. It is known that some victims of chronic insomnia do have more stage 1 sleep than is typical.

Changes within society in recent years have added to the large number of people who suffer from chronic insomnia. Light interferes with sleep, and even a bedside lamp producing low light (of only eighty lux) is enough to cause trouble. Even such dim light can suppress the release of melatonin from the pineal gland at what is usually the time of sleep onset. This sensitivity to faint light is striking. To put it in perspective, the very bright treatment lamps we use to help bring wakefulness in the morning provide ten thousand lux—that's 125 times as much as the little it takes to inhibit sleep onset!

Many of our popular electronic devices may be even worse than a low-intensity bedside lamp because the light-emitting diodes they use produce especially troublesome blue (short-wavelength) light. Mobile phones, computer screens, and tablets all can have this effect. Blue light has a greater alerting effect than longer wavelengths such as red or the yellowish light from incandescent bulbs.

Simply changing bedtime reading to an iPad from a book using a lamp can cause a shift in sleep phase. This can reset our internal clocks earlier and, in that way, delay the onset of sleepiness. The result may be increased sleepiness the next morning, as we get up to meet the demands of the world around us rather than the demands of our own internal clock. We can fortunately oppose this LED effect with a warm bath before sleep: not only does that lead to faster sleep onset, but in healthy adults it also leads to a substantial increase in delta sleep.

Chronic insomnia is harmful: life expectancy falls off steadily as the number of insomnia symptoms increases. Among same-age adult subjects with no symptoms of insomnia, 97 percent were still alive ten years later, but among those with even three insomnia symptoms only 87 percent were still alive after ten years.[3] In other words, within one decade of living with three or more symptoms of insomnia, ten more people out of every hundred lost their lives compared with every hundred people with no symptoms of insomnia.

The risk of diabetes also goes up with both insomnia and directly measured short sleep duration. Vgontzas and colleagues found a three-times higher risk of diabetes in subjects who slept less than five hours a night, compared with similar subjects who slept more than six hours a night.[4] The same study (of more than seventeen hundred adults, carefully controlled for variables that might have affected the results) showed a five-times greater risk of high blood pressure in the people who slept less than five hours a night. Almost everywhere we look, there are harmful effects on human health of too-little sleep.

Sleep specialists can usually identify the major contributors to persistent or chronic insomnia and can nearly always help improve or even restore sleep to normal. However, the harmful effects of ongoing insomnia should not be underestimated, so getting professional help when it's needed is definitely worthwhile.

The catastrophic explosion and fire in the nuclear power plant at Chernobyl, Ukraine, on April 26, 1986, was attributed to a failure of judgment by experienced but sleep-deprived plant operators. It resulted in the deaths of many incredibly brave volunteer firefighters who parachuted onto the burning and highly radioactive power plant, knowing it meant their early deaths.

A study by RAND Corporation in 2016 estimated the financial costs of sleep loss in some of the world's most advanced nations. Overall, five nations with large economies each annually lost more than 2 percent of their country's gross domestic product due to lost sleep.[5] For the United States alone that amounted to $418 billion lost due to insufficient sleep in the year 2018.

As noted in a previous chapter, another study showed how loss of REM sleep can bias our sense of risk when risk is estimated by looking at someone's facial expression. Subjects reviewed pictures of people whose expressions ranged from very friendly to very hostile.[6] After nights with limited (especially limited REM) sleep, the subjects tended to see more menace in the same faces.[7]

Widespread awareness that insomnia is undesirable has led to enormous consumption of sleeping pills. Unfortunately, frequent use of sleeping pills brings only temporary relief and, besides that, has an unfavorable effect on life expectancy.[8] Yet between 1999 and 2010, along with a 13 percent increase in US adult medical visits for insomnia, there was a 350 percent increase in prescriptions for non-benzodiazepine sleep medications among US adults and a 200 percent increase overall for sleep medicine prescription.[9]

This use was especially common among highly educated white women over the age of fifty. You'll probably agree with me that treatment not depending on such sleeping pills would be a good idea.

Professional help with insomnia often begins with a review of the patient's sleep habits, i.e. their sleep hygiene: what are her habits with regard to sleep schedule, bedtime routine, and use of alcohol, caffeine, or nicotine? These details are very clearly laid out in the useful book, *No More Sleepless Nights* by the late Peter Hauri, PhD, and Shirley Linde, PhD.[10] This book is as an excellent self-help guide. Often, adjustment of sleep-related habits is enough to relieve or even cure persistent or chronic insomnia.

When sleep professionals guide insomnia sufferers through a review of their personal habits and tactics and help weed out the ones that may be harmful, they are providing cognitive behavioral therapy for insomnia (CBT-I). CBT-I is now widely considered the first-line treatment for chronic insomnia.

Not only is it effective, but CBT is also long-lasting. Unfortunately, there is a shortage of professionals trained in its use.[11] Online computerized CBT programs are now available for self-help and have been shown to be effective. Seventy-eight percent who tried, did fully complete one such program, and twenty-five percent recovered from their chronic insomnia without further assistance.[12]

There are many CBT-I programs currently available online. Here are a few:

1. https://stellarsleep.com (from Harvard University)
2. https://www.gotosleepdoc.org (from The Cleveland Clinic)
3. https://mcpress.mayoclinic.org/living-well/think-

your-way-to-sleep-cognitive-behavioral-therapy-for-insomnia/

Insomnia sufferers often show an increased level of alertness, sometimes called a hyper-vigilant state. This condition makes it difficult for them to relax enough to allow sleep to come over them. It isn't possible to force sleep to begin, and most of us rarely need to even think about it. Once on a regular daily schedule, people with healthy sleep habits automatically begin to feel sleepy as bedtime approaches. This coincides with the appearance of predictable brain wave patterns (PGO waves). These start in the same part of the brain every night and follow an orderly progression to other predictable regions.[13] As this electrical pattern plays on, there are also recognizable changes in the body outside of the brain: breathing stabilizes and eyes slowly roll from side to side. At some point we lose the ability to have conscious thoughts, to keep track of time subconsciously, to hear any but very loud sounds, or to know if the lights go on or off. We are asleep. (An exception to this pattern is seen with new mothers, who even when asleep can detect the very faint cry of their own baby.)

Some people become very worried about their sleep problems and thus accidentally increase their level of anxiety as sleep time approaches. Because sleep starts when we're feeling warm and comfortable, safe and relaxed, bed-time anxiety can help perpetuate insomnia. One way this can show up may be what has been called sleep state misperception (also known as subjective insomnia or paradoxical insomnia). With this disorder, the insomnia sufferer may remember very long periods in bed frustrated by the belief that sleep has still not started. She may experience reverie-type thoughts: she can hear, she can appreciate changes in light brightness, and most importantly she can keep rough track of time—even for the entire night. Brain wave activity during such periods may show that she has entered stage 1 sleep, but her perception may be that she has not fallen asleep at all.

Normally stage 1 sleep occupies only about 5 percent of our nights, but in insomnia patients with hyper-alertness, this can stretch to 15 percent or even more. Once stage 2 is entered, there is normally no conscious awareness of being. It's as if our brain has turned off our self-awareness. Once a person with subjective insomnia understands the phenomenon, she is sometimes able to relax better and enter sleep more easily, but the reality of this condition is a little more complicated.

Using the power of artificial intelligence to analyze polysomnograms of patients with insomnia by three separate approaches, Andrillon and colleagues have shown that they could identify three distinctly different patterns. The results show non-overlapping patterns for 1) healthy sleepers, 2) insomnia patients without sleep state misperception, and 3) insomnia patients with sleep state misperception.[14] How to further interpret this information is not yet clear, but it is reassuring to find objective physiologic evidence that the different clinical patterns do have different and identifiable patterns of brain electrical activity.

Another difference between insomnia patients and normal sleepers was reported in early 2020 by Hermans and his colleagues.[15] They found that healthy sleepers were aware they'd fallen asleep after they'd had twenty-two minutes of uninterrupted sleep. In contrast, they found that people with insomnia were not able to recognize sleep until they had had thirty-four minutes of uninterrupted sleep. The people with sleep stage misperception were even slower to recognize that they had fallen sleep: they needed forty minutes of uninterrupted sleep. I don't know about you, but I find these differences amazing. If, for example, a person who wakes up frequently during the night and can't recognize he's been asleep until almost three quarters of an hour have passed in sleep, it's not hard to understand how he might think he's never fallen asleep at all.

I first encountered the problem of sleep stage misperception at the Cedars Sinai Sleep Clinic some years ago, when overnight sleep studies were still commonly used to evaluate chronic insomnia. My patient was an architect in his fifties who claimed that he had hardly slept at all for the preceding few months. During our interview on the morning following his overnight polysomnogram, I asked how well he had slept the previous night, during the sleep study. "You know, last night was much better than usual. I think I slept about thirty minutes." I pointed out that his brain waves showed more than five and a half hours of sleep, to which he responded with some expletives about the reliability of our sleep study. Ultimately, though, he was reassured. (Incidentally, it is common for people with chronic insomnia to sleep better when they sleep away from home.)

So insomnia is another example of good news and bad news: The bad news is that chronic insomnia carries a high price tag: not only are emotional health and even longevity compromised in individuals but whole economies suffer from lost productivity. The good news is that effective help for chronic insomnia is widely available from individual therapists, books, and online self-help programs.

10

Why Am I So Sleepy?

A very friendly 285-pound professional cowboy complained that he felt sleepy all the time, even though he allowed seven to eight hours every night for sleep. He was able to ride horseback all day at work and could tolerate working outdoors all night on horseback when necessary to protect cattle in rain and snow. After his evaluation and a diagnosis of obstructive sleep apnea (OSA), he was given a device to provide continuous positive airway pressure (CPAP) during sleep. As he left the office he said, "Doc, do you really think I'm going to use that thing?" One month later, he returned with the remark, "Doc, I'm going NOWHERE without that machine!"

Many people are sleep deprived simply because they allow too little time for sleep, as we've already noted. Others, however, feel and really are desperately sleepy even though they do allow enough time. While there are many possible causes of this too-common situation, the most common by far is OSA. In the US alone, there are at least nine million sufferers. Worldwide, the number among us who suffer from moderate to severe OSA during middle-life (age thirty to sixty-nine) is enormous. Based on the relatively stringent diagnostic criteria set forth in 2012 by the American Academy of Sleep Medicine, a careful analysis published in 2019 estimated that number to be 936 million, with prevalence exceeding half the population in certain areas if mild cases were included. The public health importance of this problem is difficult to overestimate.[1]

What is OSA? *Apnea* means a period of time without breathing. That period must be longer than ten seconds to be considered abnormal, since when we're resting, we normally pause for a few seconds between breaths. *Obstructive* refers to temporary narrowing or even complete blockage of the normal air passage from the nose (or mouth) into the lungs. Usually this happens in or just below the part of the airway called the pharynx. There, some combination of tongue, soft palate, tonsils, fat deposits in the neck, and muscle relaxation act to produce an obstructed airway.

Many factors determine whether the upper airway remains open while we're awake and after we fall asleep. It is known that many people with OSA have abnormally high muscle activity in the (pharyngeal dilator) muscles that stretch the airway open, even while they're awake.[2] This probably means that physical features of their neck would cause airway narrowing if that were not prevented by their increased awake muscle tone.[3] MRIs from the University of Pennsylvania and elsewhere show that this is often due to excess fatty tissue in the neck.[4]

As we fall asleep, tone decreases in all voluntary muscles, including these. If the increased tone is needed to keep the airway open during wakefulness, then that airway will probably collapse and cause some degree of obstruction in the upper airway as soon as we fall asleep. Recent experiments from Harvard support this idea by showing complete relief of OSA in mild cases—not from using the usual treatment of CPAP but from taking by mouth a combination of two drugs: Atomoxetine and Oxybutynin.[5] Atomoxetine increases alertness, and Oxybutynin opposes involuntary contraction of some muscles.

A more basic question is, Why does blocking the upper airway during sleep cause excessive daytime sleepiness?

Whether the upper airway is totally blocked or only partway narrowed during sleep, the brain detects a discrepancy between the effort needed to take in a breath and the amount and speed of air actually getting into the lungs. This basic alerting response is a very primitive one, needed to prevent choking. It is essentially the fight-or-flight response needed in an emergency. With airway narrowing, there is an outpouring of hormones from the adrenal glands (part of the sympathetic nervous system) and prompt changes in heart rate and blood pressure, as well as an immediate increase in the brain's alertness. Although now on alert, the brain usually does not become fully awake. Even so, the benefits of this emergency response are great: the air passage re-opens as various muscles in the neck and throat recover from their recent sleep-associated relaxation, air enters the lungs, and the body's fight-or-flight response calms down.

Unfortunately, this experience may be repeated over and over throughout the night. In order for sleep to have restorative value, it has to continue uninterrupted for at least ten minutes at a time.[6] Each time the brain is partially awakened, this ten-minute "egg-timer" has to start over. In severe OSA, this sequence (sleep, obstruct, alert, partial arousal, reopen airway, back to sleep, repeat) may happen more than one hundred times per hour of sleep. In that case, the brain may only rarely get as much as ten minutes of sleep without interruption. The result of this can be sleepiness so profound that it resembles narcolepsy.

A forty-five-year-old physician had recurrent brief lapses of alertness during lectures and while examining patients. She was known to have fallen asleep mid-sentence and have loud snoring. She admitted to waking herself occasionally with a long and very loud snore. She often had a dry mouth after sleep, and she had noticed problems with both her short-term memory and her general energy level. Her Epworth sleepiness score (a widely used estimate of chances of falling asleep under various circumstances) was 18—no different from many patients with narcolepsy (see below). She was not overweight and, except for a scalloped tongue, had a normal mouth examination. An overnight polysomnogram (PSG) confirmed severe OSA, and one observed period of REM was recorded less than fifteen minutes after she fell asleep. In the normal symphony of sleep, REM is delayed for seventy to ninety minutes after sleep onset, and SOREMPs (sleep-onset REM periods) are a hallmark of the disorder called narcolepsy. Within a few weeks of using a CPAP device, her memory lapses had stopped, her energy returned, and her snoring disappeared. Her daytime sleepiness was greatly reduced. She still fell asleep easily but no longer within one minute of lying down for sleep.

But not every patient with OSA acts sleepy.

After I gave a lecture on sleep to a group of physicians, one of them told me he was very concerned about his three-year-old daughter. During the day, she seemed entirely healthy—perhaps even hyperactive—but she snored loudly every night, keeping both parents awake. They worried that something must be dangerously wrong with her. Her health was otherwise excellent. When I examined her, enlarged tonsils were the only abnormality I could find. After they were removed, the snoring and hyperactivity disappeared. Twenty years later, she became a beautiful bride. (Frenetic daytime activity is common in young children with OSA.)

The effects of repeatedly obstructing the airway during the night go beyond excessive daytime sleepiness. Very large increases in the risks of diabetes, high blood pressure, stroke, heart attack, and early death are also results of untreated OSA. We need more evidence to understand exactly how these are all tied together, but it's far from a trivial problem. Though less than 3 percent of the US population has OSA severe enough to justify treatment, people with OSA account for almost 50 percent of all the sudden cardiac deaths occurring between midnight and 6 a.m. The level of risk is in proportion to the number of obstructive events every hour.

For those with only mild OSA, sleeping on their sides and avoiding sleeping on their back may be adequate treatment.[7] There are several devices available to help ensure that the patient doesn't accidentally roll over onto the back during sleep and they are reported to be both well tolerated and effective.[8]

Because the millions of people in this country who have OSA create a big demand for evaluation and medical care, medical insurers recognize the need for diagnoses to be made and treatment to be provided. Until recently, the usual way to diagnose OSA was to obtain a PSG in a highly specialized laboratory. Although these are labor-intensive, they are the gold standard and are still necessary for all but the most straightforward cases. PSGs include continuous measurement throughout the night of heart rate, breathing pattern, movement of the chest and abdomen, blood oxygen level, and activity of the eyes and several other muscles. More recently, it has become clear that for uncomplicated cases, a diagnosis of OSA can be made at home with simpler devices.[9]

Once a diagnosis has been confirmed, treatment can be offered in a number of ways. The most common is use of a CPAP device. The mask is connected to a quiet, portable air pressure device designed to keep the airway from closing during sleep. Modern versions of these devices are surprisingly comfortable, once adjusted and familiar. (Other treatment methods that can be used in certain patients include body-positioning devices, tonsillectomy, mandibular advancement devices or surgery, uvulo-palato-pharyngoplasty, hypoglossal nerve stimulators, and splints for the soft palate, among others.) Infrequently, oxygen is added to the incoming air to stabilize the breathing rate and depth or to compensate for other problems that reduce the oxygen level in the blood. Use of CPAP and other treatments can significantly improve the control of diabetes, difficult-to-treat high blood pressure, and certain cardiac disorders. CPAP can dramatically reduce the severe daytime sleepiness felt by many people with untreated OSA. Though not appropriate for complicated cases, the simpler methods now available for use at home in the patient's normal sleeping environment include WatchPAT,[10,11] ARES,[12,13] Apnea Link,[14,15] and others.

There is a close relationship between OSA and excessive body weight. Historically, this has been considered to be a one-way street, with high body weight causing the OSA. There is now evidence that reality is not that simple.

A fifteen-year-old boy rebelled against his father's authority, he said, by purposely overeating for several years. After school, nearly every day, he would eat an entire loaf of bread with butter and jam. When he came to an emergency room for the tenth time three years later, he had massively swollen ankles and a very flushed complexion. He was unable to stay awake during his medical interview. He was a perfect living image of "the fat boy, Joe," as described 185 years earlier in *The Pickwick Papers* by the very astute novelist Charles Dickens.[16] My patient's blood oxygen level was far below normal, and his blood carbon dioxide level was far above normal—both the result of inadequate breathing (technically, reduced alveolar ventilation). Then only eighteen years old, he was 73 inches tall and weighed 550 pounds. In addition to OSA, he had a condition we now call obesity-hypoventilation syndrome (OHS), though at the time I was responsible for his care in New York, the official term was "Pickwickian syndrome."

At that time, we couldn't understand why he was able to eat so much without feeling full the way most of us would. His appetite was not "turned off" even as he gained so much weight. The mystery was deepened by the following patient's story. Purely by chance, I cared for these two patients at the same time, more than fifty years ago.

A fifty-two-year-old bartender was admitted to an intensive care unit of a university hospital for his thirteenth time with life threatening right heart failure. He had swelling from his feet to his upper thighs and was unable to lie flat in bed. At 74 inches tall, he weighed 650 pounds and slept across two steel-framed beds for adequate support. After recovery from his acute heart failure, he was studied in the metabolic research ward. On a day when he was asked to eat as much as he could, he took in fifteen thousand calories. When I later asked if he had stopped eating because he finally felt full, he said, "Heck no. I could have eaten a lot more, but I was getting embarrassed!"

I'll bet you find this as amazing as I do. The result for him also was OSA with OHS.[17] Recent studies have shown that there are hormones, leptin and ghrelin, that help make us feel full or feel hungry, respectively. Their release by the brain changes during sleep, and sleep that's interrupted by frequent apneas may reduce appetite control by interfering with their normal release. So weight gain increases the risk of sleep apnea, and sleep apnea itself may reduce appetite control, leading to further weight gain. That's a pretty nasty positive feedback loop. As is often true in science, a closer look makes this story a little less clear: in the absence of OSA, obesity is associated with abnormally high ghrelin and elevated leptin levels. This discovery raises the possibility that there is resistance to the normal effects of leptin in obese people without OSA.[18] CPAP treatment decreases levels of both leptin and ghrelin.[19] Overall, it seems likely that hormonal control of appetite plays a role in the relationship between body weight and OSA, but our understanding is currently incomplete.

Not all people with excessive daytime sleepiness have OSA, of course. There are a few with a dramatically increased need for sleep above the usual. Some of these need only more hours of sleep to feel perfectly normal (long sleepers).[20] Others are very sleepy even after sleeping long hours at night (idiopathic hypersomnia).[21] The help of a sleep professional is needed when extra hours of sleep don't resolve abnormal sleepiness.

There are other forms of apnea that can be seen during sleep. During adjustment to high altitude, there's usually a period of several days when periodic breathing occurs and the pauses between breaths can be much longer than ten seconds. This pattern has been found during scientific studies of sleep at high altitude, though any bed partner could probably make the diagnosis without a scientific study. The reason this occurs has been clearly understood for decades and is due to changes in carbon dioxide levels in blood and spinal fluid in the first few days at a high altitude.[22]

Central sleep apnea refers in general to repeated episodes with breathing pauses, each lasting longer than ten seconds and not caused by obstruction of the airway. The pauses in breathing are caused by a temporary failure of the brain to send out breathing signals to the diaphragm and chest muscles on schedule. The basic cause of this is a misalignment in the brain's "servo-control" mechanism.[23] This normally adjusts our breathing rate and depth just enough to keep the blood level of carbon dioxide (and to a lesser degree, oxygen) very stable no matter what we're doing at the moment. Amazing though it seems, the human servo-control system is so good that the brain or spinal fluid CO2 level, as well as CO2 level in arterial blood, is normally kept at almost exactly 40 mm of mercury pressure whether we're quietly seated at a computer terminal, walking to work, or even running almost as hard as we can—when oxygen intake has increased by more than ten or even twenty times above the resting level. Wouldn't it be wonderful if we could also control our blood pressure that well?

In most cases of central sleep apnea, this misalignment of the servo mechanism is caused by slowed blood flow from the lungs to the part of the brain that contains the servo-control system responsible for adjusting our CO2 level. (That is, specifically, the medulla oblongata of the spinal cord.) This kind of sluggish blood flow can be caused by a blocked blood vessel (as in the case of a stroke) or due to weaker flow of blood from the heart (as in congestive heart failure).[24] The resulting characteristic pattern is called Cheyne–Stokes respiration and carries grave consequences. Death often follows in less than a year. Urgent medical attention is required.

It is possible to produce Cheyne–Stokes respiration artificially in an experimental animal by increasing the length of the path for arterial blood to get from the heart to the brain. Then if something reduces or increases the level of oxygen or carbon dioxide in the blood coming from the lungs, it would take longer for that altered blood to reach the brain than it normally would. When the brain's servo mechanism would try to adjust the breathing pattern to bring the blood carbon dioxide or oxygen level back to normal, it would overcorrect for the problem. Once it recognized the need for an adjustment, the breathing adjustment would go on for too long, until the slowed blood flow would bring the newly adjusted blood levels back to the medulla oblongata. That overcorrection would then cause the breathing to be either too little or too much—but again the signal would reach the brain too late and an overcorrection in the other direction would result. The result would be periods of very fast and deep breathing alternating with periods with little or no breathing—apneas. (This brilliant and simple carotid artery experiment was carried out by one of my mentors, the late Dr. Julius H. Comroe Jr.)

A ninety-one-year-old retired physician suspected he had sleep apnea. His ankles were swollen at the end of the day, and his heartbeat was quite irregular. An overnight sleep study confirmed OSA, and his EKG showed atrial fibrillation, but he also had central sleep apnea—caused by the delay of brain signals needed to regulate breathing. In his case, the sluggish blood flow was due to congestive heart failure. When treatment with a CPAP mask was provided, the obstructive events largely disappeared but the central sleep apnea became significantly worse! After a few weeks on CPAP, he was no better. Breathing support was then provided using a servo-ventilator, which triggered breathing on schedule when the brain did not.

After another month of treatment, his irregular heartbeats and ankle swelling had largely disappeared. Treatment-emergent central sleep apnea is now often recognized as a complication of treatment with CPAP. Treatment can be successful with either servo-controlled ventilation where appropriate, or simply by more prolonged use of ordinary CPAP.[25]

Changes in blood carbon dioxide that affect breathing during sleep are not limited to the hyperventilation seen at high altitude and the associated fall in blood level of CO2.

When my colleagues and I first installed a sleep laboratory at the West Los Angeles Veterans Administration Hospital, we soon found a man whose servo-controller had been dramatically affected by chronically elevated carbon dioxide level in his blood (and thus also in his spinal fluid). We knew before his sleep study that he had an abnormally high blood CO2 level (based on the elevated bicarbonate level in his venous blood). The sleep study not only confirmed the presence of OSA but it showed frighteningly long apneas. One recorded period without a breath lasted three full minutes. No known pearl diver in the world can go that long without a breath. (Skeptics may want to try—on dry land, please.) Amazing though this observation was, it was soon followed by another local record: a different patient stayed quiet without a breath for four minutes. We must note that sleep labs now have protocols to interrupt this degree of dangerous involuntary breath-holding. For any readers who want a deeper understanding of how this might occur, we offer a hint: chemical buffering capacity of the spinal fluid.

Yet another cause of periodic breathing with repeated apneas is the effect of narcotics or other central nervous system suppressing drugs, most often recreational heroin use or treatment with methadone.

Patients treated with methadone to help them recover from addictive (and far more dangerous) heroin use may not experience unusual daytime sleepiness if their dose is appropriate. Frequently, however, their sleep pattern shows prominent bursts of central apneas. Typically, these show cycles of breathe-apnea-breathe that are much shorter than those seen with the Cheyne–Stokes respirations of congestive heart failure. Unless blood oxygen levels fall to worrisome levels during the night, usually no treatment change is provided. Oxygen treatment is able to decrease the number of periodic apneas by reducing what is called "loop gain" of the breathing servo-control system, but oxygen use is limited in part by fear that the brain may have become dependent on low oxygen levels to trigger the next breath. The use of methadone (and other narcotics) suppresses the brain's responsiveness to many stimuli, including elevated carbon dioxide or low oxygen in the blood.

Excessive daytime sleepiness occurs not only from periodic interruptions of breathing during the night but from other conditions as well.

A twenty-eight-year-old sound engineer reported that he was desperately sleepy most of the time and was afraid he might lose his job. Despite three alarm clocks, he could not wake up in the mornings. His very supportive work supervisor phoned him most days to help wake him up, often more than once. He usually took a nap at work in the afternoon to keep from falling asleep involuntarily while working. Most days he had sudden episodes of muscle weakness, dropping coffee cups or pens at work (cataplexy), and he had no idea what caused those episodes. He insisted they were not caused by falling asleep or by fainting. After the diagnosis of narcolepsy was established, appropriate medical treatment with Xyrem (the sodium salt of gamma-hydroxybutyric acid) eliminated most of these attacks of cataplexy. With several timed twenty-minute naps scheduled during the day, he was able to have a near-normal level of alertness. He was the first patient I had ever treated with Xyrem, and both he and I considered the results a home run.

Narcolepsy is a condition affecting about as many people as multiple sclerosis. It causes havoc in the lives of the people it affects, until the diagnosis is discovered and effective treatment is started. Although now more often recognized during childhood, this condition was previously diagnosed most often in teen years, and sometimes even much later. Until diagnosis and treatment, these desperately drowsy people often fall asleep at school, at work, and elsewhere. Other people often consider them lazy, dullards, or slackers. They have often had trouble succeeding in school and often lost jobs. With untreated symptoms coming during the most important years of their education, the sufferers have often experienced permanently limited life prospects. People with narcolepsy can also be subject to sleep attacks that are overwhelming and totally irresistible.

Several decades ago, a twenty-seven-year-old medical student lay down on the floor and fell fast asleep in the midst of a party with about thirty other noisy students. At the time, there was no known way to definitely establish a diagnosis of narcolepsy—which was suspected—as opposed to the effects of severe sleep deprivation. Little could be done for the student at that time. Contemporary sleep specialists would obtain sleep lab studies and, if needed, could even measure the level of the important alerting hormone hypocretin in his spinal fluid.

Patients with narcolepsy also may experience hallucinations

at sleep onset or when waking up and may experience total paralysis of all voluntary muscles except the eye muscles and breathing muscles. These attacks may last less than a minute or even many minutes. Although they end without treatment, the episodes can be terrifying until they become familiar and therefore less threatening. A bizarre but related feature in some patients with narcolepsy is, as mentioned earlier, cataplexy—the sudden and brief relaxation of some or even many of the voluntary muscles in the body. These attacks may be as subtle as the drooping of an eyelid or the jaw or may involve sudden collapse to the floor—always without loss of consciousness. They are typically precipitated by an emotion, such as fear or laughter. Another frightening symptom associated with narcolepsy is hallucinations. These may occur either at sleep onset or upon arousal and may have features of psychosis. Narcolepsy is more common among people with certain inherited variants of HLA (human leucocyte antigen) genes and always requires professional help with diagnosis and treatment.

We now know that cataplexy occurs in patients with type 1 narcolepsy when the brain can't produce enough hypocretin. Hypocretin is a major hormone that supports alertness. There is a genetic component to this narcolepsy type. There is also strong evidence that narcolepsy does not become obvious until many cells within a tiny part of the brain (the suprachiasmatic nucleus) have been damaged or destroyed. Most often this damage results from an unidentified autoimmune process. Perhaps this is the reason most people in the past did not receive a diagnosis until teen or later years, even after consulting multiple physicians in vain. (Some reports claim the average delay was fifteen years, after consulting five physicians.) With better understanding of narcolepsy in the sleep medical community, its diagnosis can often be established even in young children, to their great advantage.

Hypocretin seems to function as an On-Off switch for sleep. When its secretion is impaired by narcolepsy type 1, the normal coordination of various aspects of sleep may malfunction. As we'll see, this can result in parts of the brain acting as if they're awake while other parts haven't got the message and act as if still asleep. One striking example is in patients suffering from REM sleep behavior disorder (RBD). They may not be paralyzed (as normally they would be) during even the most vivid REM dreams. (For a further exploration of this phenomenon, see the patient vignette in the following chapter.)

Other patients (with narcolepsy type 2) produce barely adequate amounts of hypocretin, but the receptors for that neurotransmitter don't function normally. A similar form of narcolepsy with cataplexy has been seen in several dog breeds studied extensively at Stanford University.

Fortunately, effective treatments for narcolepsy are now available. Some combination of scheduled brief naps, alerting medications such as armodafanil or methyphenidate, and Xyrem to control cataplexy can bring normality or at least sufficient alertness for many narcolepsy patients to function successfully at school and work.

In this chapter we've discussed the most common causes of excessive daytime sleepiness. We started with the simplest and probably most common cause: insufficient hours allowed for sleep. We then reviewed several types of sleep apnea—each one causing long periods without a breath. Switching gears, we saw how narcolepsy can play havoc with a person's employment and, by inference, also his education and life's prospects. Fortunately, we reviewed effective treatments as well.

11

Strange Things Can Happen in the Night

There's a lot of coordination in sleep. Murphy (whoever he is), states in his first law that if something can go wrong, it will[1]—and so it is with sleep. In some people, the usually flawless coordination of the unconscious, the muscular, the hormonal, the cardiovascular, and the other components of the symphony of sleep can get out of step with one another. The effects can go from amusing or embarrassing to even dangerous for the sleeper or his mate.

A seventy-one-year-old professor of nursing consulted her doctor (me) with a broken wrist and said she had no idea how it happened. She just found it when she woke up in the morning. Trying to be protective, I innocently asked if she had an abusive bed partner. She tartly denied having any bed partner. What caused her broken wrist remained a mystery, and she healed without further incident, but several years later, she came back to see me again under similar circumstances. This time, she had severe pain in the hips and pelvis, again saying she didn't know what had happened. But x-rays showed a broken pelvis—a major injury. Once again, she said that she simply woke up in bed that morning with severe pain. At the time of that visit (thirty-five years ago), I was flummoxed and couldn't reach a diagnosis. The sleep disorder I now think was the cause of her broken bones, RBD, had then been only recently described in Minneapolis and was at that time still brand new.[2]

In normal sleep, stage REM involves very active dreaming and also paralysis of all the voluntary muscles except those of the eyes and the diaphragms. This paralysis protects us because it would be dangerous to "act out" some of the scary and violent dreams of stage REM. Sometimes the paralysis fails, most often in older men but sometimes even in children. That's when nightmares in a totally unconscious sleeper can cause violent thrashing around in bed.[3] Sometimes the dreamer even gets out of bed and attacks the furniture, a wall, or even his bed partner without ever awakening. Patients with RBD have been known to hurt themselves and return to bed without any memory of the injury.[4] They may even fall down stairs and wake later in the morning wondering why they're in pain. Looking back, it seems very likely that my patient had RBD. She died a few years later of unrelated causes.

More recently, a study of almost two thousand people showed that RBD is present in just over 1 percent of the population.[5] This warns us of a coming personal and public health problem since many patients with RBD will develop Parkinson's disease and/or dementia in their later years.[6] Patients with a diagnosis of RBD will benefit from counseling about their future healthcare needs and should be enrolled in preventative treatment programs as these become available.

Many new parents are frightened to notice repeated head banging or rhythmic rocking episodes in their infants. There's usually no injury, and this startling activity leads to calm sleep (at least for the infant). The same unexpected behavior can sometimes continue into adulthood, and it seems to bring no trouble with sleep quality. That may not be true, of course, for the bed partner.

A healthy-appearing twenty-nine-year-old man reported that he awoke many mornings with a headache. His wife, a respiratory therapist, said that on many nights, she would wake to find him rocking back and forth. He would repeatedly hit his head against the back of the bed, and he always seemed to be completely asleep. After several minutes, he'd just stop and continue quietly asleep. In the morning, he never remembered his head banging, and in every other way, he seemed completely healthy. His wife was not frightened, but she did complain of lack of sleep. The man's overnight sleep study showed no other abnormalities, and he was treated successfully with a small nightly dose of a benzodiazepine sedative, Clonazepam. The end of this odd behavior was applauded, especially by his wife. There are reports of mental handicaps in some patients whose head banging continues into adulthood, but this man appeared to be intellectually intact.[7]

A much more common movement disorder that can disturb sleep is called periodic limb movements of sleep (PLMS). PLMS can occur during any non-REM stage and thus predominates in the first half of the night. The frequency and pattern of movement through time are defined by the American Academy of Sleep Medicine and can involve just one limb or even all four.[8] The movements can be very subtle or very dramatic and disturbing to the bed partner. Sleep professionals can offer medical treatments that bring relief.

Restless legs syndrome (RLS), on the other hand, is a very important cause of reduced health-related quality of life.[9] It's found mainly in adults and is more common as age increases, but it's seen also in children. Unlike PLMS, RLS involves odd symptoms or sensations that are often hard for the victim to define. Some patients describe them as creepy, crawly, pulling, or even painful. These very unpleasant feelings are worse at rest and cause limb movements that simply can't be suppressed by the patient. Movement is the only way to get relief. How it's related to PLMS is not clear. RLS is a similar movement pattern seen especially during afternoon wakeful hours but with symptoms getting more severe towards evening and then in the night. Medicines of the dopamine class often bring relief, but their use is complicated. They can make the symptoms worse and make them start earlier in the day. When it's severe, RLS can make nighttime sleep almost impossible and even force some sufferers to reschedule their sleep to daylight hours. Iron deficiency in the brain is associated with increased symptoms, and iron replacement therapy can bring at least partial relief to some.[10] I can personally report that large amounts of caffeine are a good way to have your own experience with RLS if you're so inclined. (However, I don't recommend that.)

Other failures of sleep coordination include sleepwalking, sleep eating, sleep sex, sleep headaches, loss of bladder control, and exploding head syndrome. Exploding head syndrome is a surprisingly common, usually painless, sensory neurologic event that occurs most commonly as sleep begins or ends. It is benign but may be very upsetting to the victim. Some seizure types and other unusual kinds of movement can also occur mainly or only during sleep.

An eighty-three-year-old woman admitted that she was afraid to sleep alone in her apartment, as she might open the door and go out in her sleep. She had been a sleepwalker for almost her entire life and, as a child, was once found walking outside her house by her parents. They later told her she had been fully asleep. Her personal solution after the death of her husband was to pay a companion, whose job included making sure that the front door and windows stayed locked all night long. In every other way, this woman's health was normal.

Sleepwalking arises most often from delta sleep, so it's usually in the first half of the night. Injury connected to it seems to be uncommon.

A couple came together for help after twenty-nine years of happy and stable marriage. They reported an unusual and embarrassing sleep problem that had bothered them for more than twenty years. The husband reported that almost every night around midnight, his wife would let out a terrifyingly loud scream, then roll over and continue her undisturbed sleep. He loved his wife, but his sleep was roughly jolted every night. Besides that, they were too embarrassed to take a chance on overnight visits with relatives or even stay in hotels.

I'm uncertain how to classify this woman's condition. Is it night terrors in an adult? From the husband's description, the sound seems to be made in the larynx (voice box) during air exhalation, and the timing might suggest non-REM (delta) sleep, which is typical for night terrors. In some ways it resembles catathrenia, which is usually described as a groan or moaning sound arising from sleep that does not necessarily wake the sleeper—as opposed to the bed partner.[11] But most catathrenia episodes arise from stage REM,[12] and that is seen more commonly during later hours. A different type of sound is typical of night terrors.

Typical is the abrupt arousal—usually of a child—who suddenly lets out a terrified (and terrifying) scream. The child is usually highly agitated but totally unaware of his surroundings—aware instead only of his terrifying dream. Parents are usually not able to awaken the child as he is temporarily responsive only to his brain's own internal activity and hardly at all to the environment. Incoming information from his surroundings has been largely blocked at the thalamus. All his parents can do is simply protect him from injury while he gradually calms down and returns to sleep. Although night terrors are typical of childhood, they may persist or even start in adult life.[13] In this couple's case, night terrors may have been the cause, even though there was never any evidence of fright, dreaming, or sleepwalking.

Night-time leg cramps are a very common problem of unknown cause.[14] Although they can be very painful and persistent, they are usually easily reversed by forcing the cramped muscle to stretch. Used together, the muscles that oppose the force of the cramping muscle can overcome it. When cramps occur in the calf muscles, standing at the bedside usually allows relaxation of the muscle that's in spasm.

12

Does Short Sleep Lead to Diabetes, Hypertension, and Obesity?

There's striking overlap among official United States maps showing where people get less sleep than the national average and similar maps showing where there's a lot more diabetes, more high blood pressure, more overweight bodies, and more obstructive sleep apnea. Since these four conditions are among the most expensive public health problems we have, it's worth asking why they are so closely related.[1]

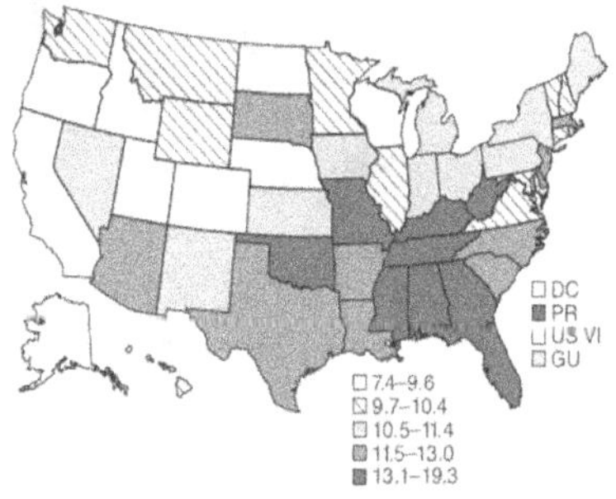

Distribution of Inadequate Sleep as Percent of US State Populations

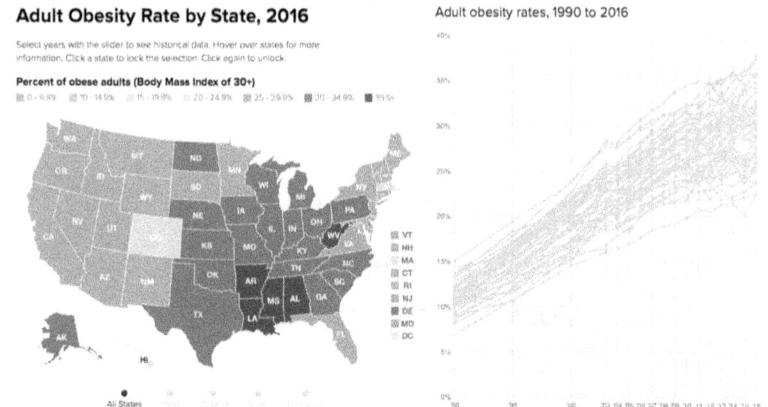

Percent of US Adults With Body Mass Index of 30 or more in 2016.
Right panel shows dramatic increase from 1990 to 2016.

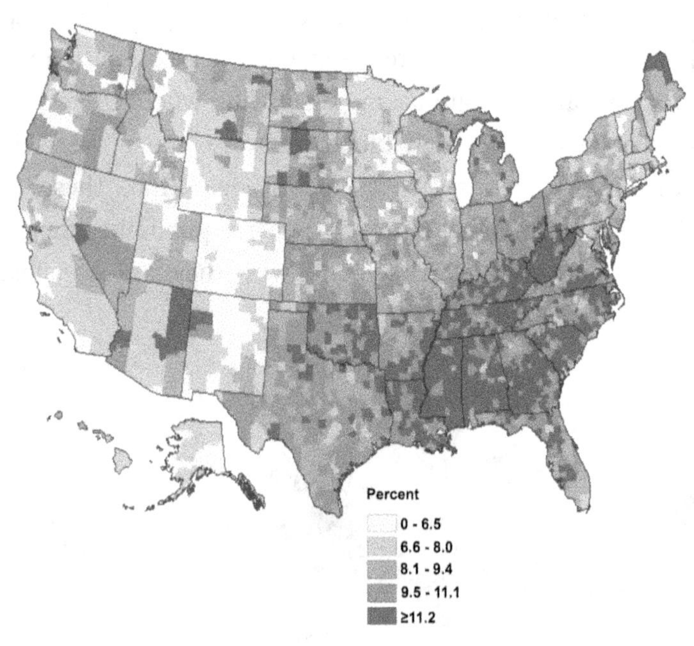

Distribution of diabetes in the USA, as Percent of Population

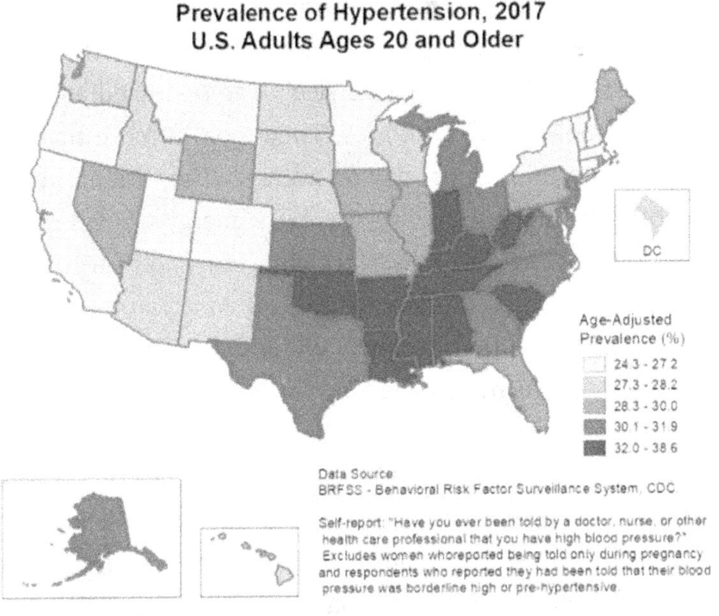

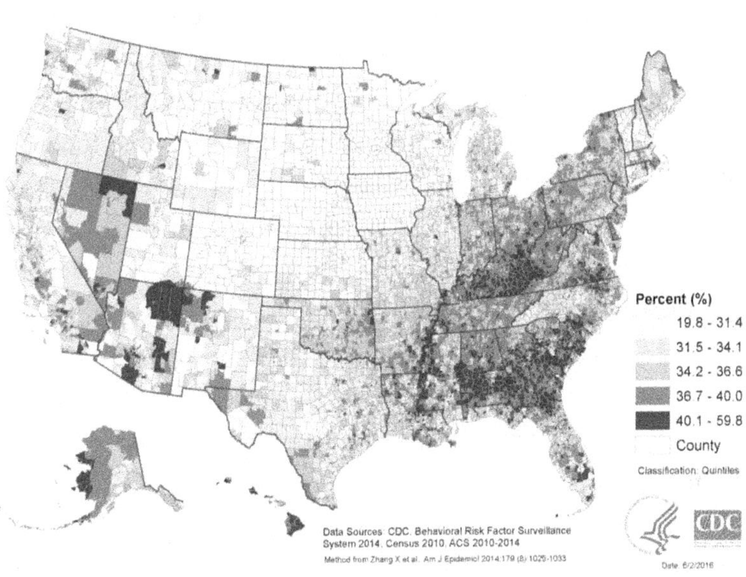

Prevalence of Obstructive Sleep Apnea (OSA) 2014

Repeatedly over the past twenty years, striking hormonal changes have been reported in people with too little sleep. Healthy adult volunteers whose sleep was restricted ate more meals and took in more calories. They took in more than five hundred extra calories per day on average. They ate more than enough extra calories to cover the extra energy needed to stay awake longer. The result was weight gain—not surprisingly. This was true especially among African Americans and more severe among men than women. Wu and colleagues reached a similar conclusion from reviewing fifteen published studies of obesity and sleep deprivation. They found that sleeping too little led to a 45 percent risk of being obese.[2] These and similar studies help explain the mysterious ability of my 650-pound patient (mentioned in chapter 10) to consume more than fifteen thousand calories in one day without feeling full.

Exactly how disruptions in our sleep result in poor health is an area of intensive study. With the discovery of a mutated version of the Clock gene in mice, scientists at Northwestern University soon found that mutation carried an increased risk of obesity compared with mice eating the very same food, but with a normal Clock gene.[3] Generally, Clock genes are known to influence daily rhythms of sleep, metabolism, and intestinal tract function.

Hints of the way this might happen had also been discovered by Spiegel and her colleagues. They showed that during a period of sleep debt, glucose tolerance decreases; that prediabetic-like condition was later repaired by a period of longer sleep.[4]

Abnormal glucose tolerance tests have long been the classic way to diagnose diabetes (though simpler methods are now available). It turns out that even fragmentation of sleep without any decrease in total sleep hours reduces our ability to keep blood sugar levels normal, and it does this by reducing the body's sensitivity to insulin. So, probably, we should not be surprised that OSA, with its frequent sleep disruption, is closely associated with diabetes.

Despite Hobson's statement that sleep is "of the brain, by the brain, and for the brain,"[5] it is now clear that this understates the much wider impact of sleep throughout the body. Even isolated normal human fat cells, for example, can't handle glucose normally after a period of sleep restriction: they show decreased insulin sensitivity.[6]

OSA is more common among both men and women who are overweight and is proportional to the degree of overweight[7] and can be reduced in severity by weight loss.[8] OSA is also found in more than half of all diabetic subjects.[9] Going even beyond that, blood sugar control in diabetic patients is worse when sleep apnea is more severe.[10] However, when CPAP is used to treat OSA, the blood sugar levels fall.[11] By withdrawing CPAP therapy from subjects with known OSA, Chopra and his colleagues found that even within one single night, blood glucose and circulating free fatty acids increased and remained above baseline levels for the entire night.[12] These are exactly the changes seen when diabetes gets out of control. It's hard to escape the conclusion that untreated OSA either causes or worsens type 2 diabetes. For any diabetics with OSA, this may be worth remembering next time they're tempted to take off their CPAP mask at night.

As if to emphasize the point, a 2020 review by Qie and colleagues showed in a large group of adults that the ten-year risk of becoming diabetic was proportional to the severity of their OSA. This was true even when the effects of obesity and percent body fat were taken into account.[13] Even mild OSA brought a 16 percent increase in that ten-year risk. Their conclusion was based on combining the results of sixteen studies involving more than thirty-three thousand subjects. During the ten years of the study, those subjects developed more than thirteen thousand cases of diabetes. The link between diabetes and OSA seems to depend on more than obesity alone: loss of sleep (due to OSA) is another very important factor.

Shift workers make up another large group of people at great risk from the combined effects of abnormal sleep, reduced control of blood sugar, and excess body weight. When our sleep hours are not in step with the cellular clocks we have in every part of our body, there is metabolic trouble. That trouble was confirmed in one monumental study of two hundred thousand nurses. Weight gain and the risk of obesity matched all too well the number of years spent working on rotating night shifts.[14] In a different meta-analysis of fifteen individual studies including more than two hundred fifty thousand people, Anothaisintawee and colleagues confirmed that shift work all by itself carried a 40 percent increase in risk of diabetes.[15] Helping us understand why this happens are the results of a study of volunteers at Harvard Medical School who were asked to sleep at times out of phase with their internal clocks: the results were increases in both blood sugar and insulin levels, as well as an increase in the stress hormone, cortisol.[16] Cortisol is part of the fight-or-flight reaction and causes a rise in blood glucose.

The almost unbelievable history of my 1999 patient who ate food adding up to fifteen thousand calories in one day (chapter 10) raised my suspicions that there was something mysterious and abnormal in his never feeling full. Since 2004, it's been known that people who allow only four hours sleep a night secrete less of the appetite-suppressing hormone leptin.[17] The problem is made even worse by a second problem also caused by inadequate sleep: an increase in ghrelin—the appetite-stimulating hormone.[18]

Overall, it is now crystal clear that short-changing ourselves of sleep brings increased hunger, increased food intake, increased body weight, and diabetes. Recurring sleep disruption leads to the same harmful metabolic consequences—whether it's caused by fewer hours for sleep, changing sleep schedules due to shift work, experimental sleep interruptions, or the effects of inadequately treated OSA. From a national point of view, this is an epidemic—an expensive and disastrous public health problem. Reader please take note: inadequate sleep can hurt you.

13

Effects of Aging on Sleep and Memory

As we get older, our need for sleep doesn't decrease, but the available evidence strongly suggests that our ability to get that sleep does decrease. What keeps us from getting the sleep we need? Several factors are at work. There are more disease-related and age-related pains in the joints, there's more health-related anxiety, there's more worry and frustration concerning family and financial security, and there's more trouble controlling the comfort of our environment.

There are also changes in our nightly sleep patterns. For example, slow-wave or delta sleep—so important in allowing memory-related fine-tuning of the developing brain and in learning at every age—gradually disappears starting at about age thirty. REM and stage 2 sleep typically continue to account for roughly 25 percent and 50 percent of each night, and stage 1 sleep may last longer with age. Since it's easy for a sleeper to confuse being in stage 1 sleep with being awake, this doubt can lead to anxiety about insomnia (sleep state misperception). See the patient vignette in chapter 9.

It's normal at all ages to be sleepy, not only at our usual

bedtime but also in the early afternoon. As our day moves on after we wake up, adenosine accumulates in the brain and circadian alertness begins to fade. As we get older, the urge to take naps increases, and so does the freedom to take naps when we feel like it. Many of us take advantage of this opportunity and usually feel more alert after even brief naps (ten to twenty minutes generally restores alertness). If the naps are too long, they can blunt the sleepiness that normally comes as evening turns into night—and that can cause trouble falling asleep at our usual bedtime. That problem is called sleep-onset insomnia. If you wander the halls of any hospital unit for depressed patients or most extended-care facilities for the elderly, you'll see many people sound asleep during the daytime. Often they're sitting in wheelchairs in the busy corridors, where they've been moved in hopes of helping them stay awake. Many of these same people have trouble falling or staying asleep at night. When that happens, they are often given sleeping pills to keep them from being noisy and disruptive when others are trying to sleep. That starts a troublesome cycle.

Because the metabolism of these sleep medicines can be very slow in the elderly, the effect is often still greater sleepiness during the next day. That results, in turn, in an even greater problem falling asleep that next night. This issue is especially difficult to handle in patients with dementia, since they also have difficulty responding to social cues regarding wake and sleep hours—even without brain-affecting drugs. Between ages twenty and thirty-nine, fewer than 2 percent of adults in the general population use sleep aids, but after age eighty years, at least three times as many do.[1]

Even without the effects of long naps or nighttime sleep medications, older people tend to have a circadian rhythm that is remarkably different from younger people's. In teenagers and young adults, sleepiness may not show up until well past midnight. That causes the expected trouble getting up for school or work the next morning. If it interferes with daytime function, this "night-owl" pattern is called delayed sleep phase syndrome. (See student vignette in chapter 4.) With increasing years, the internal clocks of most adults gradually advance so that they (we!) get sleepy earlier in the evening than they (we!) did in their younger years. During most of our adult lives, the majority of us adapt easily to a sleep pattern that fits with the timing needs of our social and working lives. But as maturity gradually becomes old age, the result can be the "lark" pattern. "Larks" tend to get sleepy and retire quite early and then awaken early. If that pattern interferes with normal social function, it is called advanced sleep phase syndrome. In the elderly, this can pose a tough challenge for their caregivers. Caregivers may not want to retire before 9 p.m. and start their day at four or five in the morning to ensure the safety of their charges. (This was a challenging problem in the case of my octogenarian friend and patient with sleepwalking described in chapter 11.) Dementia—especially common in the elderly—makes the problem even harder to manage.

Many older adults spend long months or even years largely confined within their own homes, in nursing homes, under long-term psychiatric care, or in other extended-care facilities. Except for private homes, these must usually be organized around principles of efficiency rather than around attempts to provide ideally individualized care. With advanced age, the growing instability of our internal clocks and daily rhythms makes us even more dependent than we were previously on daily exposure to strong light. Bright light, especially in the morning, is needed to keep our body rhythms aligned with the schedule of the world around us. As shown elegantly by Dr. Sonia Ancoli-Israel and her colleagues in San Diego, this disruptive pattern of aging is made worse in many institutional settings by (typically) very limited exposure to bright light during the daytime.[2,3] The result is the weakening of the pineal gland's normal rhythm that brings the release of the sleep-signaling hormone melatonin as evening sleep time approaches.

As we've noted, fewer hours of sleep also reduces the normal clearance from the brain (by the glymphatic system) of toxic waste products like beta-amyloid and the protein Tau.[4,5,6]

Buildup of these compounds within the brain is thought to contribute to early Alzheimer's dementia. Society has already seen an ominous trend of increasing dementia among the elderly,[7] so we must hope that further causes of sleep loss can be minimized. That's something you can largely control in your own life.

A great deal of research has recently helped us understand how changes in sleep of the elderly relate to changes in their brain, their mental functions, and to daily consequences. Using the tools of modern neuroscience to study how we learn, investigators have shown that sleep plays a very large role. If we think of the brain's memory as something like the hard drive storage unit of a computer system, we can understand that a certain amount of housekeeping is needed to keep the hard drive (with all our memories) neatly organized. Ideally, we'd like to file new memories temporarily in an inbox while we sort out which ones we want to keep and then move those to permanent storage files. We'd like easy access to all stored memories, but we would not want that huge library of stored memories to get in the way of immediate recall for the most important ones. If a polar bear is charging us, we don't want our brain's "flight" signals slowed down by memories of doing the breakfast dishes. That kind of daily reorganizing and filing away of our memories occurs largely during sleep.

We know that not all memories are handled in the same way and that the way any particular memory is handled changes through time. Some memories are retained only briefly (perhaps the taste of this morning's fruit juice) and fade from easy access within hours or days. Others survive the transfer from recent memory into the long-term storage parts of the brain—for easy recovery after many months or even decades (for example, the sound of tires screeching before an auto crash we may have witnessed). Most of this processing of memories also takes place during sleep.

We know that sleep becomes more fragmented as we age and that we're more easily awakened. More of our sleep is in the lighter stages (1 and 2), and we are sleeping for smaller parts of the time we're in bed (decreased sleep efficiency). However, the decreased amount of slow-wave sleep may be the most important change in terms of our ability to learn new information as we age. The number of slow waves and the associated sleep spindles (discussed in earlier chapters) decrease as we age. As they decrease, our ability to imprint new memories (largely in the hippocampus) and to transfer them later for long-term memory (especially via the thalamus into the cortex at the front of the brain) is more and more impaired compared to younger adults. Interestingly, these losses are more prominent in men (as our wives will readily attest).

Many, but not all, of the healthy elderly take daytime naps, especially men. Even though blood levels of adenosine—the substance associated with pressure to sleep—are higher in the elderly than in younger adults, current evidence suggests that this does not result in a greater overall level of sleepiness. The explanation is not certain at this time.

Another very important electrical feature of non-REM sleep that changes with age is sleep spindles. What is called the spectral power of these spindles is simply the total amount of electrical energy being used in waves at the frequency of 12-15 cycles per second. With aging, the spectral power of these spindles decreases steadily, especially as the end of each night's sleep approaches. This change is most prominent in the front part of the brain. The role of sleep spindles in processing new memory was discussed in chapter 5.

Besides the decrease with age in the spectral power of spindles during non-REM sleep, there is also a decrease in the spectral power of non-REM slow waves—also especially over the frontal cortex. Among the elderly, the slow waves of non-REM sleep are not as tall in recordings made at the surface of the scalp as they are in younger people. This means they have a lower voltage, and that, in turn, means that the firing of individual brain cells is less closely synchronized in the aged. During sleep after a study session for learning new material, slow-wave sleep promotes the transfer of new memory from the hippocampus to the cerebral cortex for long-term memory storage. This process is called consolidation. The long-term memory can then be retrieved from the cortex without any need for participation by the hippocampus (which immediately after learning serves as the short-term storage depot). However, as age causes decreased slow-wave electrical activity in the frontal cortex, the overnight transfer of new memory from the hippocampus to the cerebral cortex is reduced. The result is impaired learning.[8] To some degree, caffeine counteracts this memory impairment.[9]

Sleep is less stable in the elderly. Older people have more

changes of sleep stages during the night and more sleep-wake transitions. Proportional to this instability is the anatomic loss of cells that secrete a substance called galanin, located near the front of the brain.[10] Galanin inhibits wakefulness and so allows sleep to be better sustained.

There's an important distinction between awakenings during the night—for example when the bladder calls—as opposed to the more subtle changes we call arousals. With arousals, the sleeper is unaware of any change, but the brain waves seen with EEG recordings show a distinctive and often brief change in signals so that the (faster and less synchronized) waves briefly resemble an awake brain rather than a sleeping brain. Experiments in human volunteers and in animals show that disrupting the continuity of non-REM sleep with brief sound-induced arousals or movement can cause impaired storage of new memory into the hippocampus the next day—even though the amount of sleep and sleep efficiency (as currently measured in most sleep laboratories) are unchanged.[11] Pity the unfortunate New Yorkers or Chicagoans trying to learn while living right by the noisy subway lines (as I used to)! And think of those with untreated OSA, whose sleep may be interrupted by brief arousals as often as one hundred times per hour or even more. With age, many people need various medicines that can unintentionally interrupt slow-wave sleep.

Other experiments with volunteers have shown the opposite effect: increasing the spectral power of slow-wave, non-REM sleep improves their next-day ability to learn—that is, to encode new memories into the hippocampus. Such experiments were performed using either low-voltage rhythmic electrical signals applied to the head or using gentle rocking beds tuned to the frequency of the slow waves of sleep. The result was an increase in the spectral power of slow-wave sleep together with improved memory.[12]

It's not known whether aging changes in the brain decrease the ability to recall successfully stored old memories. It is known, though, that sleeping before an attempt to recall old memories does increase the chances of success—at least in young adults.

As we noted earlier, the gradual age-related deterioration of non-REM sleep is worse in men. Why then do women report more sleep complaints than their age-peer men? The answer is not yet fully known.

14

Especially for Women

At all ages, women sleep more hours than men.[1,2] Even so, women feel more sleep-deprived than men except when they're between twenty and twenty-four years old.[3] Between ages twenty-five and twenty-nine, more than a quarter of women surveyed reported struggling with sleep more often than three nights a week. Common problems with sleep in women are the same as those in men: OSA,[4] RLS,[5] and insomnia—especially in mid-life,[6] but there are differences as well. Sleep disturbances—particularly in women of color—have been reviewed by Heilermann.[7]

Compared with boys, girls have an earlier decline in slow-wave sleep, starting once they have menstrual periods.[8] As progesterone increases each month, towards mid-cycle, they experience more time awake after sleep has started. Problems with menses are associated with a two- to three-times increase of insomnia.

During pregnancy, problems with sleep increase—much as you'd expect from the increasing weight, bigger abdomen, and elevated diaphragm due to the enlarged uterus, hormonal changes, and also the anxieties related to becoming a new parent. OSA increases, central sleep apnea increases, and so does RLS. Fortunately, CPAP treatment for OSA is safe in pregnancy.[9] Opposite to the sleep disturbance seen when menstrual periods begin, breastfeeding has the effect of substantially increasing slow-wave sleep for the new mother.[10]

The hot flashes of menopause also disturb sleep, and many menopausal women report having severe insomnia.[11] Hormone replacement therapy helps decrease these hot flashes and has regained the confidence of medical authorities some years after the Women's Health Initiative initially questioned its prolonged use.[12] Oher approaches to treatment include antidepressants and related medicines.

Another factor playing a role in disturbed sleep doesn't apply only to women but probably affects women more than men simply because they have more insomnia. That is the use of digital communication devices in the late evening. That habit has, of course, become widespread all over the world. Television, mobile phone screens, iPads, digital-book readers, and similar devices can expose our eyes to high-energy (i.e., short wavelength) blue light starting just as sleep time approaches. While the entertainment and teaching value of these devices is wonderful, the effect on our sleep cycle is not.[13] For people who have no insomnia, we can offer congratulations: their sleep rhythms are strong enough to resist a challenge that lots of other people can't handle. For those with sleep-onset insomnia, however, it is worth thinking about whether exposure to blue light before bedtime is part of their problem. Blue light exposure might be keeping their pineal gland from its normal release of melatonin at bedtime.[14,15]

15

Sleep and the Heart

Some years ago, I gave a talk to the pulmonary specialists at Cedars Sinai Medical Center entitled "Does the Heart Care If We Snore?" There was already a lot of evidence that the heart really should care. It was already known at that time that high blood pressure, irregular heartbeats (including that all-too-common type called atrial fibrillation), and worsening of heart failure were all unexpectedly common in people with sleep disturbances, including just too few hours. In the vast majority of people with high blood pressure—probably far more than 95 percent—no cause of their high blood pressure had yet been found, even after extensive (and expensive) evaluation. But recently, it's become obvious that many patients with "essential" hypertension also have OSA. (Estimates vary from 30 percent to 85 percent of such people, far beyond the much lower numbers with OSA in the general population.) With effective treatment of OSA, blood pressure falls. But no one knew what it was about improved sleep that could reduce blood pressure and what it was about OSA that could raise blood pressure. An intriguing clue was offered in the 1975 book by Herbert Benson, MD, and Miriam Z. Klipper titled *The Relaxation Response.*[1]

Benson, then an academic psychiatrist at Harvard Medical School, thought that the many stressful events of modern life (especially in big cities) must trigger a sense of danger, increased alertness, and anxiety in most of us, probably many times every day. The normal human response to stress is to turn on the fight-or-flight response. That primitive response to danger was absolutely necessary to the survival of our distant ancestors who needed an immediate and automatic response to the presence of predators and other enemies. In our lives, just as then, that response would increase attention and focus, muscle tone, heart and breathing rates, and would raise blood pressure—all thanks to the release of stress hormones like epinephrine, norepinephrine, and cortisol. A large-scale analysis from China (based on records from more than one hundred fifty thousand people) found that medically diagnosed anxiety came along with an 18 percent increased risk of high blood pressure.[2] Since hypertension is one of the leading causes of death worldwide, that points to an important problem in public health.[3] In prehistoric times, each such event would lead to a prompt resolution: either a successful fight or flight or else the end of the individual. But today, there is usually no such quick solution to most of the anxiety-provoking situations, and the hyper-vigilant state may go on for a long time once it's triggered. That may bring a high cost to our health.

Benson then went on to describe various forms of relaxation practiced in different cultures throughout history. Maybe you won't be surprised that they are all very similar and involve quiet time, being nearly motionless, and focusing the mind on an object or a sound. In people experienced in the form of relaxation response called Transcendental Meditation, he found jaw-dropping biological responses: Oxygen consumption per minute (a good measure of overall metabolic rate) fell within just a few minutes to numbers lower than seen under any other non-sick condition—even lower than seen during deep sleep. Blood lactate levels also fell by nearly half within thirty minutes. Who cares? you might ask, but previous studies of patients with high levels of anxiety and panic attacks done at Washington University School of Medicine in Saint Louis found that blood lactate levels were abnormally high in those patients. Besides that, panic attacks could be produced by giving lactate by vein—not only in these patients but also in some subjects with no history of either high anxiety or panic attacks. Similar findings have been reported by a number of other scientists since that time.[4,5] So, Transcendental Meditation and similar forms of relaxation can be expected to reduce chronic anxiety and acute anxiety by reducing the blood lactate level in some—perhaps most—people. On the other hand, disrupted sleep can activate the sympathetic nervous system with dangerous results, as we shall now see.

Finding and treating problems that cause reduced or impaired sleep could have a big impact on the public's health—and yours. The most common sleep disorder known to cause heart problems is OSA. Before we turn to that very common problem, though, let's return to the title of my previous lecture, "Does The Heart Care If We Snore?" Snoring all by itself is associated with mental decline in the elderly.[6] It's not trivial in younger adults, either: snoring medical students are more likely to fail exams than their colleagues matched for similar age, sex, and body mass index.[7] In pregnancy, snoring is associated with increased blood pressure.[8] It is a risk factor for cardiovascular disease in women.[9] It is a risk factor for type 2 diabetes.[10] It contributes in a very big way to the lethality of other well-known cardiovascular risk factors such as obesity, high cholesterol, and high blood pressure. Compared with healthy people, those with both snoring and cardiovascular risk factors have seven times the normal death rate.[11]

So, the heart does care if we snore, but it also cares if we have OSA. When atrial fibrillation is stopped using electrical shock (cardioversion), those with untreated OSA are twice as likely to relapse into atrial fibrillation within one year compared with those whose OSA is treated.[12]

I referred previously to atrial fibrillation as an all-too-common arrhythmia because it's associated with blood clots thrown from the heart to various parts of the body, including the brain—often with dangerous strokes resulting. In patients with left-sided congestive heart failure, mortality in the next two years was related to both the severity of their heart failure (measured by enlargement of the heart's left atrium) and to the severity of OSA, measured by apnea-hypopnea index (AHI). No matter how severe their heart failure, people with only mild OSA had less than 20 percent risk of dying in the next two-plus years. On the other hand, if they had severe sleep apnea with severe heart failure, nearly 80 percent of them failed to stay alive for more than eight months.[13]

Four to eight years after they were enrolled in the Wisconsin Sleep Heart Health Study, people had developed high blood pressure at a rate that was proportional to the severity of OSA when they entered the study. Without OSA at the beginning, they had only a 20 percent chance of having high blood pressure four years later. But if they had more than mild OSA at the start, that risk was almost four times as great, similar to the risk of death among patients in the study of OSA and heart failure that we just mentioned.[14]

Looking for OSA in folks who've had a stroke is definitely not reassuring: more than half of all people with a first stroke do have OSA. Among those who've also had a second stroke, the number is 80 percent with OSA! It's beginning to sound like it may be more than the heart that cares if we snore or have OSA: how about the brain?[15]

In 2007, doctors at the Mayo Clinic found even more reasons that the heart will care if we have OSA. They checked patient records in more than five hundred consecutive overnight sleep studies and found OSA in well over half. In the families of people with OSA, fatal heart disease was more than twice as common as it was in the other families.[16]

Fortunately, there is evidence that treatment helps. In twenty-five people with both coronary artery disease (CAD) and worse-than-mild OSA who were treated with CPAP, "only" 25 percent of them had a cardiovascular event in the next seven years. Among twenty-nine other people who had both OSA and CAD but refused treatment for OSA, almost 60 percent had such an event in the same time, suggesting that CPAP treatment cut the risk by half or more. Statistical analysis showed it to be less than 1 percent likely that this result was due only to random chance.[17]

Although it has yet to be proven conclusively that CPAP reduces overall mortality from OSA, there is reason to believe it does. Before Sullivan's development of CPAP in 1981, the standard treatment for life-threatening OSA was to place a permanent opening in the neck below the larynx.[18] This procedure is called tracheostomy, and a study at Stanford showed that it did indeed save lives.[19] A later extensive study from Canada that was intended to corroborate the benefits of CPAP failed at first to show any statistically significant survival benefit.[20] Closer analysis suggested that among the sleep apnea patients whose CPAP was truly adequate and did verifiably reduce the (AHI), that benefit was demonstrated. As of this writing, I'm not aware of any more definitive study in subjects with OSA, except for proven benefits in a special group of patients who have both OSA and severe chronic obstructive pulmonary disease with chronically elevated levels of carbon dioxide in their blood.[21]

Still, if you or someone dear to you snores or has long breathing pauses during sleep, you may be able to make a very important difference in that person's life by helping them get medical attention for that problem.

16

How Can This Book Help You Improve Your Sleep?

What makes a person become a student of sleep, and what prepared me to tackle the challenge of writing this book? It was hard to forget the nineteen-year-old hospital patient who couldn't stay awake while I interviewed him. No one then understood the connection between his great weight, his sleepiness, and his terrible problems with his heart and lungs.

As a consultant in chest medicine, I noticed that sleeping patients often displayed long periods without taking a breath but sometimes couldn't understand why. The opportunity soon arose to attend a wonderful course on polysomnography (overnight sleep studies) given by faculty from Stanford University and others, and it was too tempting to ignore. Other courses on sleep taught at the annual meetings of the American Thoracic Society and the American College of Chest Physicians followed, and ultimately, I became a diplomate of the American College of Physicians/Sleep Medicine. As I began to evaluate and treat patients referred for help with their sleep problems, to review and interpret polysomnograms, and to be invited to give talks about sleep issues to various medical and public audiences, one thing became increasingly obvious: there is a great thirst in our society to better understand what is happening inside us when we sleep and why things sometimes go wrong in ways we don't understand. It occurred to me (time for a genuine Midwestern blush!) that I was well qualified to help.

Unusual for medical people, I had received actual training in delivering medical and scientific lectures; as a professor and director of programs to train specialists in pulmonary medicine, I had delivered hundreds of lectures (without too many students snoring noticeably) and had reviewed many of the known sleep problems with my own patients who suffered from them. Encouraged by the COVID epidemic, the time seemed ripe to retire from active practice and make time available. That is how I came to write this book.

Many of us wish we could sleep better. Maybe that's even the main reason you chose to read this book. So now that we've seen many of the ways that our personal sleep patterns can give us something less than full satisfaction, what can we do about our problems?

Whatever your sleep issues may be, a good place to start is to create consistent sleep habits. Determine what is the earliest time you must get out of bed during your typical week's schedule. Get up at that time every single day, but allow for one day to sleep in later if you so choose. So that you're not constantly checking the clock (or more likely your cell phone) to see how much time you have left to sleep, set an alarm and stick to it. This will help mitigate feelings of anxiety and panic that can arise from counting down the hours until you have to wake up (and save your brain from a flood of blue light from your cell phone screen in the middle of the night). Getting up when the alarm goes off (resist the urge to hit that Snooze button!) will help anchor your body-clock rhythms, which will make it easier to get up at that time in the long run. Once you are awakened by your alarm, exposing yourself to bright light will further help set your body clock to match society's demands.

For most of us, the natural length of sleep we need per night is a little longer than eight hours. Some people need several hours more while others do fine with several hours less. If you feel rested and well with a different amount, you'll probably do well to stick with what works best for you. To determine what time to turn off the lights for sleep, count backwards from the time you have to get up in the morning for however many hours of sleep you need to feel your best. For example, if you have to get up at 6 a.m., and you need nine hours to feel well rested, then make sure you are in bed with the lights out by 9 p.m.

If you have a consistent sleep schedule and are still sleepier than you think you should be, it's time to do some additional investigating. Can you identify any factors that could be disturbing your sleep hours? Are you snoring? Do you have leg or arm movements in your sleep? Do you stop breathing often during the night? Even if these seem infrequent to you, and you're not aware of them arousing you during the night (you may need help from a bed partner or, if you sleep alone, find a way to record audio and/or video of yourself sleeping), you'll need professional help from a sleep specialist to check them out. They will likely order an overnight sleep study and possibly one or more blood tests to check for your body's iron supply.

Do you have sudden and overwhelming periods of sleepiness during the day? Do you experience cataplexy, the occasional and abrupt involuntary relaxation of muscles without losing consciousness? If either is true, then it's time to see a sleep specialist.

If you have more than a few days of trouble falling asleep or staying asleep, and you're more of the DIY type, the book *No More Sleepless Nights* by Peter Hauri and Shirley Linde can help you review all the factors in your own life that can help—or interfere—with routinely satisfying and restorative sleep. If you still need help after that, try the links in chapter 9 to online self-directed CBT-I (cognitive behavioral therapy for insomnia). Most sleep clinics and many MDs and other psychotherapists offer personalized CBT to help with chronic insomnia.

If you decide to see a sleep specialist for unexpected or troubling behavior during the night, you will be served best by providing them all the information you can about the odd behavior you're experiencing. Both falling asleep and waking up bring very large changes in the electrical and chemical background in the brain, and unusual experiences can occur, especially at those times. Things like sleep paralysis and hallucinations can initially be very frightening, but reassurance usually comes with a diagnosis and treatment.

If your dreams are especially disturbing or frequently peculiar, it's worth seeking help from a therapist or sleep specialist. How dreams occur and some insight into their significance were described in chapter 6.

Sleep has a very strong influence on our ability to learn new information and also to perform as athletes. To be the best student you can be, it's important to heed the information presented in chapter 5, where the price of all-nighters on learning was highlighted. Many of the interactions between sleep and sports were reviewed in chapter 7. Paying attention to them can help you be a better (and safer) athlete, no matter whether you're a professional or a weekend warrior and no matter which sport is your favorite.

If you are prone to depression or think you may be bipolar, it's important to be on the lookout for worsening sleep. That's a time to get help without delay. Self-help is probably not the best first step in that situation. Therapists can recommend ways to combat severe depression and help you avoid sleep-related episodes of bipolar disorder.

What about other unusual experiences during sleep? Recall the woman described in chapter 11 who could not remember how she had fractured her pelvis during the previous night's sleep. She was almost certainly in very deep sleep in part of her brain, yet clearly awake enough elsewhere in her brain to leave her bed and somehow fall hard enough to sustain a major fracture and then she found her way back to bed for the rest of the night without ever waking up. For anything resembling this kind of puzzling experience, professional help is needed.

Whatever your reason for taking the time to read this book, know that you're in good company. As more information has become available, public interest in sleep has grown substantially. If you do not feel rested, and even a week or two with eight hours a night doesn't make you feel well rested, it's time to consult with a sleep specialist. Whatever the problems you may be having with your own sleep, you can feel assured that well-trained men and women are available all over this country (and in much of the world) to help you with proven and effective treatments for most of the known sleep disorders.

HOW TO FIND HELP:

There are now specialists in sleep medicine in large cities across the US, and some also hold office hours in smaller nearby communities. Most sleep medicine specialists are also trained as pulmonary specialists, neurologists, psychiatrists, internists, family practitioners, or pediatricians, while others are anesthesiologists, dentists, or surgeons. Several national organizations now provide information and further help to the public, including the American Academy of Sleep Medicine, American Sleep Apnea Association, Restless Legs Foundation, Sleep Foundation, and others. There are similarly capable specialists in sleep available in many nations worldwide.

Postscript

In this book, we have surveyed the field of sleep and how our bodies, brains, and our very survival interact with this "time off" from our awake daily lives. We've seen how widespread this pattern of daily rest is across an amazingly broad range of living creatures and how the electrical signals of our brains during sleep are organized into repeating patterns through each night in a way that strongly resembles the musical patterns of a symphony.

With the help of more than twenty brief patient vignettes from my own personal practice, we've seen how Murphy's First Law can sometimes play havoc with people's sleep and show up in unexpected ways in their daytime lives. Although this is not intended as a textbook of medical treatments, we have referred to the main ways treatment is available for many (of the now more than one hundred recognized) sleep disorders.

Because dreams are such a prominent (and sometimes troubling) feature of sleep, we've reviewed how dreams are created in the brain, and what's been learned over the past five thousand years or so about their significance and meaning.

And because the lives of people who are young today are likely to last many years longer than most lives did in the past, many (especially young) people now alive will probably need to continue working later in their lives than their ancestors did. They will need to continue learning too, as work will also change. Because sleep plays such a crucial role in maintaining the ability to learn, we've taken a look at what's currently known about how to keep our learning abilities working well.

I hope you, dear reader, enjoy this survey of one-third of your life as much as I have enjoyed learning enough to write it.

H. Kenneth Fisher MD
Los Angeles

Acknowledgments

More than sixty-five years ago, Thurlo B. Thomas* taught my Carleton College class that saltwater crabs could keep time through the night. Later, M. Henry Williams Jr., MD,* vividly pointed out the interesting connections between sleep and respiratory medicine at Bronx Municipal Hospital, Albert Einstein College of Medicine, New York. Eliot Phillipson MD, and John Severinghaus, MD,* originally kindled my interest in the science of sleep through their research seminars at the Cardiovascular Research Institute of University of California, San Francisco. Phillip Westbrook, MD, nurtured that interest through weekly sleep conferences at Cedars Sinai Medical Center, Los Angeles, over a number of years. Added to these fundamental guideposts were the fascinating and troubling personal stories told by patients of the West Los Angeles Veterans Hospital (where the enthusiasm of my colleague and friend Adrian J. Williams, MD, was contagious), and subsequently in my private practice over several decades. Herbert S. Gross Pharm D, MD,* kindled my interest in changes in the electrical power of brain waves during sleep. Colleagues in Bronx, New York, Los Angeles and Beverly Hills, California, Casper, Wyoming, and Austin, Texas, referred most of the patients whose stories help illuminate some of the sleep issues discussed in this book. A number of friends and colleagues have made helpful suggestions and comments that decreased the book's shortcomings. My thanks to each of them: Kay Kolderie White, Ken Sherman, Sandy Blakeslee, David Meltzer, MD, Anson Levine, PhD, Susan Harris, PhD, Jochen Haber, PhD, Carrie Chassin, Magda Waingrow, Matthew Elgart, PhD, Seymour Feshbach, PhD,* Alexander Astin, PhD,* Jay Miller, Pierino Teti, Sherman Pearl, Ralph Shapira, JD, Hugh Ford, James Scott, Frank Baker,* Norm Beegun, JD, Rebecca Hughes, Paul Loeb, Nan Kalish, Alan Goodman, JD, Chris Smith of SciWheel Inc., Amy Espiritu of Printland, William Solberg, DDS,* Becky Novelli, Chuck Rosenberg, JD, Phebe Berkowitz Tanners, Judith Sanford, Joan Morganstern, Bill and Nancy Boyarski, Dianne Gard, and others I may have omitted by error (and therefore owe an apology).

The sense of humor so vital to the conquest of life's challenges is kept alive by monthly video conferences with my sons Michael B. Fisher, Joshua B. Fisher, JD, and Hugh E. Fisher, PhD, further laced with the bringing-to-earth good judgment of their wives Anne and Maria. My special thanks to Elaine Fisher Goldberg who found time and energy in retirement from Cornell University to provide innumerable and expert early editorial suggestions and corrections with sisterly love and thought, all without damaging my ego beyond repair. Additional suggestions, plus the chutzpah and stamina needed to write this book stem from the support of my life partner and love, personal poet laureate and cook extraordinaire, Judith Roedelheimer Pacht.

At Torchflame Books, Betty Turnbull, Teri Rider, Jori Hanna, and Chelsea Robinson were unfailingly supportive, competent, knowledgeable, and helpful.

To each, my profound thanks and appreciation. The remaining faults are entirely my own.

H. Kenneth Fisher, MD,
Los Angeles
*of blessed memory

Notes

1. The Overture to Sleep (and how this book can help you)

1. Guy Bloch et al., "Time is Honey: Circadian Clocks of Bees and Flowers and How Their Interactions May Influence Ecological Communities," *Philosophy Transactions of the Royal Society B: Biological Sciences* 372, no. 1734 (2017): https://royalsocietypublishing.org/doi/10.1098/rstb.2016.0256.
2. Monica Kraft and Richard J. Martin, "Chronobiology and Chronotherapy in Medicine," *Disease-a-Month* 41, no. 8 (1995): 506–575.
3. Osamu Hayaishi and Hitoshi Matsumura, "Prostaglandins and Sleep," *Advances in Neuroimmunology* 5, no. 2 (1995): 211–216.

2. What's Happening in the Brain When We Sleep?

1. William Shakespeare, *Macbeth* (London: William Jaggard, 1623), 2.2.47–52.
2. Doris Moser et al., "Sleep Classification According to AASM and Rechtschaffen & Kales: Effects on Sleep Scoring Parameters," *Sleep* 32, no. 2 (2009): 139–149.
3. F. J. Mullin and Nathaniel Kleitman, "Variations in Threshold of Auditory Stimuli Necessary to Awaken the Sleeper," *American Journal of Physiology* 123, no. 2 (1938): 477–481.
4. Pablo L. Cardozo et al., "Synaptic Elimination in Neurological Disorders," *Current Neuropharmacology* 17, no. 11 (2019): 1071–1095.
5. Aurora A. Perrault et al., "Whole-Night Continuous Rocking Entrains Spontaneous Neural Oscillations with Benefits for Sleep and Memory," *Current Biology* 29, no. 3 (2019): 402–411.
6. Madeleine Grigg-Damberger et al., "The Visual Scoring of Sleep and Arousal in Infants and Children," *Journal of Clinical Sleep Medicine* 3, no. 2 (2007): 201–240.
7. Eli Robins et al., "Quantitative Histochemical Studies of the Morphogenesis of the Cerebellum. II. Two Beta-Glycosidases," *Journal of Neurochemistry* 8 (November 1961): 96–104.
8. Ashura Williams Buckley et al., "Rapid Eye Movement Sleep Percentage in Children with Autism Compared with Children with Developmental Delay and Typical Development," *Archives of Pediatric & Adolescent Medicine* 164, no. 11 (2010): 1032–1037.

9. Eugene Aserinsky and Nathaniel Kleitman, "Regularly Occurring Periods of Eye Motility, and Concomitant Phenomena, During Sleep," 1953. *Science* 118, no. 3062 (1953): 273–274.
10. Eugene Aserinsky, "The Discovery of REM Sleep," *Journal of the History of the Neurosciences* 5, no. 3 (1996): 213–227.
11. Dean Burnett, *The Idiot Brain: A Neuroscientist Explains What Your Head Is Really Up To* (Toronto, Ontario: HarperCollins, 2016), 112.

3. How Long Do We Really Need for Sleep?

1. A. M. Williamson and Anne-Marie Feyer, "Moderate Sleep Deprivation Produces Impairments in Cognitive and Motor Performance Equivalent to Legally Prescribed Levels of Alcohol Intoxication," *Occupational & Environmental Medicine* 57, no. 10 (2000): 649–655.
2. William C. Dement, *The Promise of Sleep* (New York: Delacorte Press, Random House, Inc, 1999), 3.
3. Jeffrey M. Jones, "In U.S., 40% Get Less Than Recommended Amount of Sleep: Hours of Sleep Similar to Recent Decades, but Much Lower than in 1942," *Gallup*, December 19, 2013, https://news.gallup.com/poll/166553/less-recommended-amount-sleep.aspx.
4. "2003 Sleep in America Poll," *National Sleep Foundation*, March 10, 2003, https://www.thensf.org/wp-content/uploads/2021/03/2003-SleepPollExecSumm.pdf.
5. "Science: Cave Men," *TIME*, July 18, 1938, https://time.com/archive/6759335/science-cave-men/.
6. William C. Dement and Christopher Vaughan, *The Promise of Sleep* (New York: Dell Publishing Co., 1999), 69.
7. Renata Pellegrino et al., "A Novel BHLHE41 Variant is Associated with Short Sleep and Resistance to Sleep Deprivation in Humans," *Sleep* 37, no. 8 (2014):1327–1336.
8. Jeffrey S. Durmer and David F. Dinges, "Neurocognitive Consequences of Sleep Deprivation," Seminars in Neurology 25, no. 1 (2005): 117–129.
9. Phoebe Weston, "10,000 Naps a Day: How Chinstrap Penguins Survive on Microsleeps," *Guardian*, November 30, 2023, https://www.theguardian.com/environment/2023/nov/30/rough-sleepers-how-chinstrap-penguins-survive-on-micronaps-aoe.
10. Daniel F. Kripke et al., "Mortality Associated with Sleep Duration and Insomnia," *Archives of General Psychiatry* 59, no. 2 (2002): 131–136.
11. Christopher P. Landrigan et al., "Effects of the Accreditation Council for Graduate Medical Education Duty Hour Limits on Sleep, Work Hours, and Safety," *Pediatrics* 122, no. 2 (2008): 250–258.
12. Giuseppe Iacomino et al., "Circulating miRNA are Associated with Sleep Duration in Children/Adolescents," *Experimental Physiology* 105, no. 2 (2020): 347–356.

13. Arlet Nedeltcheva et al., "Insufficient Sleep Undermines Dietary Efforts to Reduce Adiposity," *Annals of Internal Medicine* 153, no. 7 (2010): 435–441.
14. Arlet Nedeltcheva et al., "Insufficient Sleep Undermines Dietary Efforts to Reduce Adiposity," *Annals of Internal Medicine* 153, no. 7 (2010): 435–441.
15. Jana Husse et al., "Circadian Clock Genes *Per1* and *Per2* Regulate the Response of Metabolism-Associated Transcripts to Sleep Disruption," *PLoS One* 7, no. 12 (2012): e52983, https://journals.plos.org/plosone/article?id=10.1371/journal.pone.0052983.
16. Hermann Nabi et al., "Awareness of Driving While Sleepy and Road Traffic Accidents: Prospective Study in GAZEL Cohort," *BMJ* 333, no. 7558 (2006): 75.
17. Norman Ohler, *Blitzed,* trans. Shaun Whiteside (United Kingdom: Penguin Books, 2017).
18. Arianna Huffington, *The Sleep Revolution: Transforming Your Life, One Night at a Time* (New York: Harmony Books, 2016), 266.

4. Your Body Has Clocks

1. C. Richardson et al., "A Randomised Controlled Trial of Bright Light Therapy and Morning Activity for Adolescents and Young Adults with Delayed Sleep-Wake Phase Disorder," *Sleep Medicine* 45 (May 2018): 114–123.
2. Andrew Herxheimer and Keith J. Petrie, "Melatonin for the Prevention and Treatment of Jet Lag," *Cochrane Database of Systematic Reviews* 2 (April 2002): CD001520, https://www.cochranelibrary.com/cdsr/doi/10.1002/14651858.CD001520/full.
3. Matthew Walker, *Why We Sleep: Unlocking the Power of Sleep and Dreams* (New York: Scribner, 2017), 97.
4. Jennifer A. Mohawk et al., "Central and Peripheral Circadian Clocks in Mammals," *Annual Review of Neuroscience* 35, (July 2012): 445–462.
5. Jennifer Cable et al., "Sleep and Circadian Rhythms: Pillars of Health—A Keystone Symposia Report," *Annals of the New York Academy of Sciences* 1506, no. 1 (2021): 18–34.
6. Rajindra P. Aryal et al., "Macromolecular Assemblies of the Mammalian Circadian Clock," *Molecular Cell* 67, no. 5 (2017): 770–782.
7. Takashi Ebisawa, "Circadian Rhythms in the CNS and Peripheral Clock Disorders: Human Sleep Disorders and Clock Genes" *Journal of Pharmacological Sciences* 103, no. 2 (2007):150–154.
8. Derk-Jan Dijk and Simon N. Archer, "PERIOD3, Circadian Phenotypes, and Sleep Homeostasis," *Sleep Medicine Reviews* 14, no. 3 (2010): 151–160.
9. Christopher M. Depner et al., "Mistimed Food Intake and Sleep Alters 24-Hour Time-of-Day Patterns of the Human Plasma Proteome," *Proceedings of the National Academy of Sciences USA* 115, no. 23 (2018): E5390–99.
10. J. Allan Hobson, *Sleep* (New York: Scientific American Library, 1989), 2–4.

11. Annika L. A. Nichols et al., "A Global Brain State Underlies *C. elegans* Sleep Behavior," Science 356, no. 6344 (2017): eaam6851, https://www.science.org/doi/10.1126/science.aam6851.
12. Jesus Lopez-Minguez et al., "Late Dinner Impairs Glucose Tolerance in MTNR1B Risk Allele Carriers: A Randomized, Cross-over Study," *Clinical Nutrition* 37, no. 4 (2018): 1133–1140.
13. Andrew W. McHill et al., "Later Circadian Timing of Food Intake is Associated with Increased Body Fat," *American Journal of Clinical Nutrition* 106, no. 5 (2017): 1213–1219.
14. M. Garaulet et al., "Timing of Food Intake Predicts Weight Loss Effectiveness," *International Journal of Obesity London* 37, no. 4 (2013): 604–611.
15. Sharon A. Chung et al., "Sleep and Health Consequences of Shift Work in Women," *Journal of Women's Health* 18, no. 7 (2009): 965–977.

5. Sleep, Memory, and Learning

1. Lynda Gratton and Andrew Scott, *The 100-Year Life: Living and Working in an Age of Longevity* (London: Bloomsbury Publishing, 2016), 67–97.
2. George Markowsky, "Information Theory," in *Encyclopedia Brittanica,* updated August 30, 2024, https://www.britannica.com/science/information-theory/Classical-information-theory.
3. Guilherme Testa-Silva et al., "High Bandwidth Synaptic Communication and Frequency Tracking in Human Neocortex," *PLoS Biology* 12, no. 11 (2014): https://journals.plos.org/plosbiology/article?id=10.1371/journal.pbio.1002007.
4. Richard P. Feynman, *Surely You're Joking, Mr. Feynman! (Adventures of a Curious Character)* (New York: W. W. Norton, 1985).
5. Helen Shen, "Portrait of a Memory," *Scientific American Mind* 29, no. 3 (2018) 21.
6. Julia S. Rihm et al., "Reactivating Memories During Sleep by Odors: Odor Specificity and Associated Changes in Sleep Oscillations," *Journal of Cognitive Neuroscience* 26, no. 8 (2014):1806–1818.
7. Stuart M. Fogel et al., "How to Become an Expert: A New Perspective on the Role of Sleep in the Mastery of Procedural Skills," *Neurobiology of Learning and Memory* 125 (November 2015): 236–248.
8. Timothy K. Leonard et al., "Sharp Wave Ripples During Visual Exploration in the Primate Hippocampus," *Journal of Neuroscience* 35, no. 44 (2015): https://www.jneurosci.org/content/35/44/14771.
9. Matthew Walker, *Why We Sleep: Unlocking the Power of Sleep and Dreams* (New York: Scribner, 2017).

6. Sleep and Dreams

1. Genesis 20:1-18.
2. Marcel Proust, *Remembrance of Things Past* (A la Recherche du Temps Perdues) (New York: Random House, 1934).
3. Genesis 41:46-57.
4. Rosalind D. Cartwright, *The Twenty-Four Hour Mind: The Role of Sleep and Dreaming in Our Emotional Lives* (Oxford, UK: Oxford University Press, 2012).
5. Sigmund Freud, *The Interpretation of Dreams* (Die Traumdeutung) (Vienna: Franz Deuticke, 1899).
6. J. Allan Hobson, *Dreaming: A Very Short Introduction* (Oxford, UK: Oxford University Press; 2002) 15–31.
7. Philip R. Gehrman et al., "Sleep Diaries of Vietnam War Veterans with Chronic PTSD: The Relationships Among Insomnia Symptoms, Psychosocial Stress, and Nightmares," *Behavioral Sleep Medicine* 13, no. 3 (2015): 255–264.
8. M. de Boer et al., "The Spectral Fingerprint of Sleep Problems in Post-Traumatic Stress Disorder," *Sleep* 43, no. 4 (2020): https://academic.oup.com/sleep/article/43/4/zsz269/5614711.
9. Aurore A. Perrault et al., "Whole-Night Continuous Rocking Entrains Spontaneous Neural Oscillations with Benefits for Sleep and Memory," *Current Biology* 29, no. 3 (2019): 402–411.
10. William Shakespeare, *Macbeth* (London: William Jaggard, 1623), 2.2.49–51.
11. Ryan Bottary et al., "Fear Extinction Memory is Negatively Associated with REM Sleep in Insomnia Disorder," *Sleep* 43, no. 7 (2020): https://academic.oup.com/sleep/article/43/7/zsaa007/5717136?.
12. Rosalind D. Cartwright, *The Twenty-Four Hour Mind: The Role of Sleep and Dreaming in Our Emotional Lives* (Oxford, UK: Oxford University Press, 2012), 49–71.
13. John F. Gottlieb et al., "Meta-Analysis of Sleep Deprivation in the Acute Treatment of Bipolar Depression," *Acta Psychiatrica Scandinavica* 143, no. 4 (2021): 319–327.
14. Allison G. Harvey et al., "Treating Insomnia Improves Mood State, Sleep, and Functioning in Bipolar Disorder: A Pilot Randomized Controlled Trial," *Journal of Consulting and Clinical Psychology* 83, no. 3 (2015): 564–577.
15. Eti Ben Simon et al., "Overanxious and Underslept," *Nature Human Behavior* 4, no. 1 (2020): 100–110.
16. Sara Dallaspezia and Francesco Benedetti, "Sleep Deprivation Therapy for Depression," *Current Topics in Behavioral Neurosciences* 25, (2015): 483–502.

7. Sleep and Athletic Performance

1. Arianna Huffington, *The Sleep Revolution: Transforming Your Life, One Night at a Time* (New York: Penguin Random House, 2016), 266.
2. Emily Kroshus et al., "Wake Up Call for Collegiate Athlete Sleep: Narrative Review and Consensus Recommendations from the NCAA Interassociation Task Force on Sleep and Wellness," *British Journal of Sports Medicine* 53, no. 12 (2019): 731–736.
3. Melanie Knufinke et al., "Effects of Natural Between-Days Variation in Sleep on Elite Athletes' Psychomotor Vigilance and Sport-Specific Measures of Performance," *Journal of Sports Science & Medicine* 17, no. 4 (2018): 514–524.
4. Houda Daaloul, et al., "Effects of Napping on Alertness, Cognitive, and Physical Outcomes of Karate Athletes," *Medicine & Science in Sports & Exercise* 51, no. 2 (2019): 338–345.
5. Austin Anderson et al., "Circadian Effects on Performance and Effort in Collegiate Swimmers," *Journal of Circadian Rhythms* 16, no. 8 (2018): https://jcircadianrhythms.com/articles/10.5334/jcr.165.
6. Dominic Fitzgerald et al., "The Influence of Sleep and Training Load on Illness in Nationally Competitive Male Australian Football Athletes: A Cohort Study Over One Season," *Journal of Science and Medicine in Sport* 22, no. 2 (2019): 130–134.
7. Gregory W. Kirschen et al., "The Impact of Sleep Duration on Performance Among Competitive Athletes: A Systematic Literature Review," *Clinical Journal of Sport Medicine* 30, no. 5 (2020): 503–512.
8. T. Q. Chen et al., [Association between speed and endurance performance with sleep duration in children and adolescents] (article in Chinese), *Beijing Da Xue Xue Bao Yi Xue Ban* 50, no. 3 (2018): 429–435.
9. Anthony W. Blanchfield et al., "The Influence of an Afternoon Nap on the Endurance Performance of Trained Runners," *European Journal of Sport Science* 18, no. 9 (2018): 1177–1184.
10. Tristan Martin et al., "Sleep Habits and Strategies of Ultramarathon Runners," *PLoS One* 13, no. 5 (2018): https://journals.plos.org/plosone/article?id=10.1371/journal.pone.0194705.
11. Shannon O'Donnell et al., "The Influence of Match-Day Napping in Elite Female Netball Athletes," *International Journal of Sports Physiology and Performance* 13, no. 9 (2018): 1143–1148.
12. Dorothea Dumuid et al., "Relationships Between Older Adults' Use of Time and Cardio-Respiratory Fitness, Obesity and Cardio-Metabolic Risk: A Compositional Isotemporal Substitution Analysis," *Maturitas* 110 (April 2018): 104–110.
13. Matthew A. Tucker et al., "The Relative Impact of Sleep and Circadian Drive on Motor Skill Acquisition and Memory Consolidation," *Sleep* 40,

no. 4 (2017): https://academic.oup.com/sleep/article/40/4/zsx036/3765296.

14. Daniel Kahneman, *Thinking, Fast and Slow* (New York: Farrar, Straus and Giroux, 2011).
15. Matthew D. Milewski et al., "Chronic Lack of Sleep is Associated with Increased Sports Injuries in Adolescent Athletes," *Journal of Pediatric Orthopaedics* 34, no. 2 (2014): 129–133.

8. Sleep and the "Aha!" Moment

1. Juliana Yordanova et al., "Covert Reorganization of Implicit Task Representations by Slow Wave Sleep," *PLoS One* 4, no. 5 (2009): https://journals.plos.org/plosone/article?id=10.1371/journal.pone.0005675.
2. Roumen Kirov et al., "Labile Sleep Promotes Awareness of Abstract Knowledge in a Serial Reaction Time Task," *Frontiers in Psychology* 6 (September 2015): https://www.frontiersin.org/journals/psychology/articles/10.3389/fpsyg.2015.01354/full.
3. Jean-Baptiste Eichenlaub et al., "The Nature of Delayed Dream Incorporation ('Dream-Lag Effect'): Personally Significant Events Persist, but Not Major Daily Activities or Concerns," *Journal of Sleep Research* 28, no. 1 (2019): https://onlinelibrary.wiley.com/doi/10.1111/jsr.12697.
4. Saskia van Liempt et al., "Impact of Impaired Sleep on the Development of PTSD Symptoms in Combat Veterans: A Prospective Longitudinal Cohort Study," *Depression and Anxiety* 30, no. 5 (2013): 469–474.
5. Delphine Oudiette et al., "REM Sleep Respiratory Behaviours Match Mental Content in Narcoleptic Lucid Dreamers," *Scientific Reports* 8, no. 1 (2018): https://www.nature.com/articles/s41598-018-21067-9.
6. Anita D'Anselmo et al., "Creativity in Narcolepsy Type 1: The Role of Dissociated REM Sleep Manifestations," *Nature and Science of Sleep* 12 (December 2020): https://www.dovepress.com/creativity-in-narcolepsy-type-1-the-role-of-dissociated-rem-sleep-mani-peer-reviewed-fulltext-article-NSS.

9. Why Can't I Sleep?

1. William Shakespeare, *Macbeth* (London: William Jaggard, 1623), 2.2.55.
2. Christer Hublin et al., "Heritability and Mortality Risk of Insomnia-Related Symptoms: A Genetic Epidemiologic Study in a Population-Based Twin Cohort," *Sleep* 34, no. 7 (2011): 957–964.
3. Lars E. Laugsand et al., "Insomnia and the Risk of Incident Heart Failure: A Population Study," *European Heart Journal* 35, no. 21 (2014): 1382–1393.
4. Alexandros N. Vgontzas et al., "Insomnia with Objective Short Sleep

Duration is Associated with Type 2 Diabetes: A Population-Based Study," *Diabetes Care* 32, no. 11 (2009): 1980–1985.

5. Marco Hafner et al., "Why Sleep Matters—The Economic Costs of Insufficient Sleep: A Cross-Country Comparative Analysis," *Rand Health Quarterly* 6, no. 4 (2017): 11.
6. Andrea Goldstein-Piekarski et al., "Sleep Deprivation Impairs the Human Central and Peripheral Nervous System Discrimination of Social Threat," *Journal of Neuroscience* 35, no. 28 (2015): 10135–10145.
7. Anna Alkozei et al., "Chronic Sleep Restriction Affects the Association Between Implicit Bias and Explicit Social Decision Making," *Sleep Health* 4, no. 5 (2018): 456–462.
8. Jae-Won Choi et al., "Use of Sedative-Hypnotics and Mortality: A Population-Based Retrospective Cohort Study," *Journal of Clinical Sleep Medicine* 14, no. 10 (2018): 1669–1677.
9. Earl S. Ford ES, et al., "Trends in Outpatient Visits for Insomnia, Sleep Apnea, and Prescriptions for Sleep Medications Among US Adults: Findings from the National Ambulatory Medical Care Survey 1999-2010," *Sleep* 37, no. 8 (2014): 1283–1293.
10. Peter Hauri and Shirley Linde, *No More Sleepless Nights* (New York: John Wiley & Sons, 1996).
11. Wendy Troxel and Daniel Buysse, "Primary Care Intervention for Primary Insomnia," *Journal of Primary Health Care* 5, no. 1, Editorial (2013): 4.
12. Sammy K. Cheng and Janine Dizon, "Computerised Cognitive Behavioral Therapy for Insomnia: A Systematic Review and Meta-Analysis," *Psychotherapy and Psychosomatics* 81, no. 4 (2012): 206–216.
13. J. Allan Hobson, *Sleep* (New York: Scientific American Library, 1989), 2–4.
14. Thomas Andrillon et al., "Revisiting the Value of Polysomnographic Data in Insomnia: More Than Meets the Eye," *Sleep Medicine* 66 (February 2020): 184–200.
15. Lieke W. A. Hermans et al., "Modeling Sleep Onset Misperception in Insomnia," *Sleep* 43, no. 8 (2020): https://academic.oup.com/sleep/article/43/8/zsaa014/5721963?.

10. Why Am I So Sleepy?

1. Adam V. Benjafield et al., "Estimation of the Global Prevalence and Burden of Obstructive Sleep Apnoea: A Literature-Based Analysis," *Lancet Respiratory Medicine* 7, no. 8 (2019): 687–698.
2. W. S. Mezzanotte et al., "Waking Genioglossal Electromyogram in Sleep Apnea Patients Versus Normal Controls (A Neuromuscular Compensatory Mechanism)," *Journal of Clinical Investigation* 89, no. 5 (1992): 1571–1579.
3. Pedro R. Genta et al., "Upper Airway Collapsibility is Associated with Obesity and Hyoid Position," *Sleep* 37, no. 10 (2014): 1673–1678.

4. C. D. Turnbull et al., "Relationships Between MRI Fat Distributions and Sleep Apnea and Obesity Hypoventilation Syndrome in Very Obese Patients," *Sleep and Breathing* 22, no. 3 (2018): 673–681.
5. Luigi Taranto-Montemurro et al., "Effects of the Combination of Atomoxetine and Oxybutynin on OSA Endotypic Traits," *Chest Journal* 157, no. 6 (2020): 1626–1636.
6. R. Downey and M. H. Bonnet, "Performance During Frequent Sleep Disruption," *Sleep* 10, no. 4 (1987): 354–363.
7. Simon Joosten et al., "Supine Position Related Obstructive Sleep Apnea in Adults: Pathogenesis and Treatment," *Sleep Medicine Reviews* 18, no. 1 (2014): 7–17.
8. Jolien Beyers et al., "Treatment of Sleep-Disordered Breathing with Positional Therapy: Long-Term Results," *Sleep and Breathing* 23, no. 4 (2019): 1141–1149.
9. Sharon De Cruz, Michael R. Littner, and Michelle R. Zeidler, "Home Sleep Testing for the Diagnosis of Obstructive Sleep Apnea—Indications and Limitations," *Seminars in Respiratory and Critical Care Medicine* 35, no. 5 (2014): 552–559.
10. Ji Ho Choi et al., "Validating the Watch-PAT for Diagnosing Obstructive Sleep Apnea in Adolescents," *Journal of Clinical Sleep Medicine* 14, no. 10 (2018): 1741–1747.
11. Stephen D. Pittman et al., "Using a Wrist-Worn Device Based on Peripheral Arterial Tonometry to Diagnose Obstructive Sleep Apnea: In-Laboratory and Ambulatory Validation," *Sleep* 27, no. 5 (2004): 923–933.
12. Katherine M. Sharkey et al., "Validation of the Apnea Risk Evaluation System (ARES) Device Against Laboratory Polysomnography in Pregnant Women at Risk for Obstructive Sleep Apnea Syndrome," Journal of Clinical Sleep Medicine 10, no. 5 (2014): 497–502.
13. Djordje Popovic et al., "Validation of Forehead Venous Pressure as a Measure of Respiratory Effort for the Diagnosis of Sleep Apnea," *Journal of Clinical Monitoring and Computing* 23, no. 1 (2009): 1–10.
14. Hui Chen et al., "Evaluation of a Portable Recording Device (ApneaLink) for Case Selection of Obstructive Sleep Apnea," *Sleep and Breathing* 13, no. 3 (2009): 213–219.
15. Florian Stehling et al., "Validation of the Screening Tool ApneaLink in Comparison to Polysomnography for the Diagnosis of Sleep-Disordered Breathing in Children and Adolescents," *Sleep Medicine* 37 (September 2017): 13–18.
16. M. H. Kryger, "Fat, Sleep, and Charles Dickens: Literary and Medical Contributions to the Understanding of Sleep Apnea," *Clinics in Chest Medicine* 6, no. 4 (1985): 555–562.
17. Babak Mokhlesi et al., "Evaluation and Management of Obesity Hypoventilation Syndrome. An Official American Thoracic Society Clinical Practice

Guideline," *American Journal of Respiratory and Critical Care Medicine* 200, no. 3 (2019): e6–e24.

18. Zuleyha Bingol et al., "Leptin and Adiponectin Levels in Obstructive Sleep Apnea Phenotypes," *Biomarkers in Medicine* 13, no. 10 (2019): 865–874.
19. I. A. Harsch et al., "Leptin and Ghrelin Levels in Patients with Obstructive Sleep Apnoea: Effect of CPAP Treatment," *European Respiratory Journal* 22, no. 2 (2003): 251–257.
20. Sanjay R. Patel et al., "Sleep Characteristics of Self-Reported Long Sleepers," *Sleep* 35, no. 5 (2012): 641–648.
21. David Landzberg and Lynn Marie Trotti, "Is Idiopathic Hypersomnia a Circadian Rhythm Disorder?" *Current Sleep Medicine Reports* 5, no. 4 (2019): 201–206.
22. Klaus Mees Richard de la Chaux, "Polygraphy of Sleep at Altitudes Between 5300 m and 7500 m During an Expedition to Mt. Everest (MedEx 2006)," *Wilderness & Environmental Medicine* 20, no 2 (2009): 161–165.
23. Jeremy E. Orr et al., "Pathogenesis of Central and Complex Sleep Apnoea," *Respirology* 22, no. 1 (2017): 43–52.
24. K. A. Franklin et al., "Hemodynamics, Cerebral Circulation, and Oxygen Saturation in Cheyne-Stokes Respiration," *Journal of Applied Physiology* 83, no. 4 (1997): 1184–1191.
25. Dongquan Liu et al., "Trajectories of Emergent Central Sleep Apnea During CPAP Therapy," *Chest Journal* 152, no 4 (2017): 751–760.

11. Strange Things Can Happen in the Night

1. Arthur Bloch, *Murphy's Law and Other Reasons Why Things Go Wrong* (Los Angeles: Price/Stern/Sloan Publishers, 1978).
2. Carlos H. Schenck and Mark W. Mahowald, "REM Sleep Behavior Disorder: Clinical, Developmental, and Neuroscience Perspectives 16 Years After its Formal Identification in SLEEP," *Sleep* 25, no. 2 (2002): 120–138.
3. Erik K. St. Louis and Bradley F. Boeve, "REM Sleep Behavior Disorder: Diagnosis, Clinical Implications, and Future Directions," *Mayo Clinic Proceedings* 92, no. 11 (2017): 1723–1736.
4. Stuart J. McCarter et al., "Factors Associated with Injury in REM Sleep Behavior Disorder," *Sleep Medicine* 15, no. 11 (2014): 1332–1338.
5. José Haba-Rubio et al., "Prevalence and Determinants of Rapid Eye Movement Sleep Behavior Disorder in the General Population," *Sleep* 41, no. 2 (February 2018): https://academic.oup.com/sleep/article/41/2/zsx197/4690595?.
6. Ronald B. Postuma et al., "Risk and Predictors of Dementia and Parkinsonism in Idiopathic REM Sleep Behaviour Disorder: A Multicentre Study," *Brain* 142, no. 3 (2019): 744–759.
7. M. F. Mendez and A. Mirea, "Adult Head-Banging and Stereotypic Movement Disorders," *Movement Disorders* 13, no 5 (1998): 825–828.

8. Wiebke Hermann et al., "Asymmetry of Periodic Leg Movements in Sleep (PLMS) in Parkinson's Disease," *Journal of Parkinson's Disease* 10, no. 1 (2020): 255–266.
9. Richard P. Allen et al., "Restless Legs Syndrome: Diagnostic Criteria, Special Considerations, and Epidemiology. A Report from the Restless Legs Syndrome Diagnosis and Epidemiology Workshop at the National Institutes of Health," *Sleep Medicine* 4, no. 2 (2003): 101–119.
10. Narong Simakajornboon et al., Periodic Limb Movements in Sleep and Iron Status in Children," *Sleep* 26, no. 6 (2003): 735–738.
11. Jorge Iriarte et al., "Sound Analysis of Catathrenia: A Vocal Expiratory Sound," *Sleep and Breathing* 15, no. 2 (2011): 229–235.
12. Panagis Drakatos et al., "Catathrenia, a REM Predominant Disorder of Arousal?" *Sleep Medicine* 32 (April 2016): 222–226.
13. Waldemar Szelenberger et al., "Sleepwalking and Night Terrors: Psychopathological and Psychophysiological Correlates," *International Review of Psychiatry* 17, no. 4 (2005): 263–270.
14. Hubert Maisonneuve et al., "Prevalence of Cramps in Patients over the Age of 60 in Primary Care: A Cross Sectional Study," *BMC Family Practice* 17, no. 1 (2016): https://bmcprimcare.biomedcentral.com/articles/10.1186/s12875-016-0509-9.

12. Does Short Sleep Lead to Diabetes, Hypertension, and Obesity?

1. Sirimon Reutrakul and Eve Van Cauter, "Sleep Influences on Obesity, Insulin Resistance, and Risk of Type 2 Diabetes," *Metabolism Clinical and Experimental* 84 (July 2018): 56–66.
2. Yili Wu et al., "Sleep Duration and Obesity Among Adults: A Meta-Analysis of Prospective Studies," *Sleep Medicine* 15, no. 12 (2014): 1456–1462.
3. Clare Milliken, "The Rhythm of Sleep," *Northwestern Magazine,* Winter 2022, https://magazine.northwestern.edu/features/sleep-and-circadian-biology-and-health/.
4. K. Spiegel et al., "Impact of Sleep Debt on Metabolic and Endocrine Function," *Lancet* 354. no 9188 (1999): 1453–1459.
5. J. Allan Hobson, *Sleep* (New York: Scientific American Library, 1989), 2–4.
6. Josiane L. Broussard et al., "Impaired Insulin Signaling in Human Adipocytes after Experimental Sleep Restriction: A Randomized, Crossover Study," *Annals of Internal Medicine* 157, no. 8 (2012): 549–557.
7. M. Melanie Lyons et al., "Global Burden of Sleep-Disordered Breathing and its Implications," *Respirology* 25, no. 7 (2020): 690–702.
8. Almudena Carneiro-Barrera et al., "Effect of an Interdisciplinary Weight Loss and Lifestyle Intervention on Obstructive Sleep Apnea Severity: The INTERAPNEA Randomized Clinical Trial," *JAMA Network Open* 5, no. 4

(2022): https://jamanetwork.com/journals/jamanetworkopen/fullarticle/2791455.

9. Sirimon Reutrakul and Eve Van Cauter, "Sleep Influences on Obesity, Insulin Resistance, and Risk of Type 2 Diabetes," *Metabolism Clinical and Experimental* 84 (July 2018): 56–66.
10. Renee S. Aronsohn et al., "Impact of Untreated Obstructive Sleep Apnea on Glucose Control in Type 2 Diabetes," *American Journal of Respiratory and Critical Care Medicine* 181, no. 5 (2010): 507–513.
11. Babek Mokhlesi et al., "Effect of One Week of CPAP Treatment of Obstructive Sleep Apnoea on 24-Hour Profiles of Glucose, Insulin, and Counter-Regulatory Hormones in Type 2 Diabetes," *Diabetes, Obesity and Metabolism* 19, no. 3 (2017): 452–456.
12. Swati Chopra et al., "Obstructive Sleep Apnea Dynamically Increases Nocturnal Plasma Free Fatty Acids, Glucose, and Cortisol During Sleep," *Journal of Clinical Endocrinology & Metabolism* 102, no. 9 (2017): 3172–3181.
13. Ranran Qie et al., "Obstructive Sleep Apnea and Risk of Type 2 Diabetes Mellitus: A Systematic Review and Dose-Response Meta-Analysis of Cohort Studies," *Journal of Diabetes* 12, no. 6 (2020): 455–464.
14. An Pan et al., "Rotating Night Shift Work and Risk of Type 2 Diabetes: Two Prospective Cohort Studies in Women," *PLoS Medicine* 8, no. 12 (2011): https://journals.plos.org/plosmedicine/article?id=10.1371/journal.pmed.1001141.
15. Thunyarat Anothaisintawee et al., "Sleep Disturbances Compared to Traditional Risk Factors for Diabetes Development: Systematic Review and Meta-Analysis," *Sleep Medicine Reviews* 30 (December 2016): 11–24.
16. Frank A. J. L. Scheer et al., "Adverse Metabolic and Cardiovascular Consequences of Circadian Misalignment," *PNAS USA* 106, no. 11 (2009): 4453–4458.
17. Karine Spiegel et al., "Leptin Levels are Dependent on Sleep Duration: Relationships with Sympathovagal Balance, Carbohydrate Regulation, Cortisol, and Thyrotropin," *Journal of Clinical Endocrinology & Metabolism* 89, no. 11 (2004): 5762–5771.
18. Eve Van Cauter et al., "Metabolic Consequences of Sleep and Sleep Loss," *Sleep Medicine* 9, Supplement 1 (September 2008): S23–S28.

13. Effects of Aging on Sleep and Memory

1. Nazanin Abolhassani et al., "Ten-Year Trend in Sleeping Pills Use in Switzerland: The CoLaus Study," *Sleep Medicine* 64 (December 2019): 56–61.
2. Sonia Ancoli-Israel et al., "Increased Light Exposure Consolidates Sleep and Strengthens Circadian Rhythms in Severe Alzheimer's Disease Patients," *Behavioral Sleep Medicine* 1, no. 1 (2003): 22–36.

3. B. B. Lovell et al., "Effect of Bright Light Treatment on Agitated Behavior in Institutionalized Elderly Subjects," *Psychiatry Research* 57, no. 1 (1995): 7–12.
4. Helene Benveniste et al., "Glymphatic System Function in Relation to Anesthesia and Sleep States," *Anesthesia & Analgesia: Neuroscience and Neuroanesthesiology* 128, no. 4 (2019): 747–758.
5. Ehsan Shokri-Kojori et al., "β-Amyloid Accumulation in the Human Brain After One Night of Sleep Deprivation," *PNAS USA* 115, no. 17 (2018): 4483–4488.
6. Helene Benveniste et al., "The Glymphatic System and Waste Clearance with Brain Aging: A Review," *Gerontology* 65, no. 2 (2019): 106–109.
7. Maria Skaalum Peterson at al., "Trend in the Incidence and Prevalence of Dementia in the Faroe Islands," *Journal of Alzheimer's Disease* 71, no. 3 (2019): 969–978.
8. Andrew W. Varga et al., "Effects of Aging on Slow-Wave Sleep Dynamics and Human Spatial Navigational Memory Consolidation," *Neurobiology of Aging* 42 (June 2016): 142–149.
9. Daniel Borota et al., "Post-Study Caffeine Administration Enhances Memory Consolidation in Humans," *Nature Neuroscience* 17, no. 2 (2014): 201–203.
10. Alicia Garcia-Falgueras et al., "Galanin Neurons in the Intermediate Nucleus (InM) of the Human Hypothalamus in Relation to Sex, Age, and Gender Identity," *Journal of Comparative Neurology* 519, no. 15 (2011): 3061–3084.
11. Christopher P. et al., "Spatial Learning and Memory Deficits Following Exposure to 24 Hours of Sleep Fragmentation or Intermittent Hypoxia in a Rat Model of Obstructive Sleep Apnea," *Brain Research* 1294 (October 2009): 128–137.
12. Aurore A. Perrault et al., "Whole-Night Continuous Rocking Entrains Spontaneous Neural Oscillations with Benefits for Sleep and Memory," *Current Biology* 29, no. 3 (2019): 402–411.E3.

14. Especially for Women

1. Edward O. Bixler et al., "Women Sleep Objectively Better than Men and the Sleep of Young Women is More Resilient to External Stressors: Effects of Age and Menopause," *Journal of Sleep Research* 18, no. 2 (2009): 221-228.
2. Sarah A. Burgard and Jennifer A. Ailshire, "Gender and Time for Sleep among U.S. Adults," *American Sociological Review* 78, no. 1 (2013): 51–69.
3. Andrea N. Goldstein-Piekarski et al., "Sex, Sleep Deprivation, and the Anxious Brain," *Journal of Cognitive Neuroscience* 30, no. 4 (2018): 565–578.
4. Alison Wimms et al., "Obstructive Sleep Apnea in Women: Specific Issues and Interventions," *Biomed Research International* 2016 (September 2016): https://onlinelibrary.wiley.com/doi/10.1155/2016/1764837.

5. Jessica M. Baker and Albert Y. Hung, "Movement Disorders in Women," *Seminars in Neurology* 37, no. 6 (2017): 653–660.
6. Martica H. Hall et al., "Insomnia and Sleep Apnea in Midlife Women: Prevalence and Consequences to Health and Functioning," *F100 Prime Reports* 7, no. 63 (2015): https://s3-eu-west-1.amazonaws.com/science-now.reports/f1000reports/files/9008/7/63/article.pdf.
7. MarySue V. Heilermann et al., "Factors Associated with Sleep Disturbance in Women of Mexican Descent," *Journal Advanced Nursing* 68, no. 10 (2012): 2256–2266.
8. Fiona C. Baker et al., "Age-Related Differences in Sleep Architecture and Electroencephalogram in Adolescents in the National Consortium on Alcohol and Neurodevelopment in Adolescence Sample," *Sleep* 39, no. 7 (2016): 1429-1439.
9. Dennis Oyiengo et al., "Sleep Disorders in Pregnancy," *Clinics in Chest Medicine* 35, no. 3 (2014): 571–587.
10. D. M. Blyton et al., "Lactation is Associated with an Increase in Slow-Wave Sleep in Women," *Journal of Sleep Research* 11, no. 4 (2002): 297–303.
11. P. Proserpio et al., "Insomnia and Menopause: A Narrative Review on Mechanisms and Treatments," *Climacteric* 23, no. 6 (2020): 539–549.
12. Santiago Palacios, et al. "Hormone Therapy for First-Line Management of Menopausal Symptoms: Practical Recommendations," *Women's Health* (London) 15 (August 2019): https://journals.sagepub.com/doi/10.1177/1745506519864009.
13. Sarah L. Appleton et al., "Waking to Use Technology at Night, and Associations with Driving and Work Outcomes: A Screenshot of Australian Adults," *Sleep* 43, no. 8 (2020): https://academic.oup.com/sleep/article/43/8/zsaa015/5727773?.
14. Ari Schechter et al., "Blocking Nocturnal Blue Light for Insomnia: A Randomized Controlled Trial," *Journal of Psychiatric Research* 96 (January 2018): 196–202.
15. S. A. R. Mortazavi et al., "Blocking Short-Wavelength Component of the Visible Light Emitted by Smartphones' Screens Improves Human Sleep Quality," *Journal of Biomedical Physics & Engineering* 8, no. 4 (2018): 375–380.

15. Sleep and the Heart

1. Herbert Benson and Miriam Z. Klipper, *The Relaxation Response* (New York: Avon Books, 1975).
2. Yu Pan et al., "Association Between Anxiety and Hypertension: A Systematic Review and Meta-Analysis of Epidemiological Studies," *Neuropsychiatric Disease and Treatment* 11 (April 2015): 1121–1130.
3. Rafael Hernández-Hernández et al. "Results of May Measurement Month 2018 Campaign in Venezuela," *European Heart Journal Supplements: Journal of the European Society of Cardiology* 22 (Suppl H) (August 2020): H135–138.

4. L.A. Papp et al., "Arterial Blood Gas Changes in Panic Disorder and Lactate-Induced Panic," *Psychiatry Research* 28, no. 2 (1989): 171–180.
5. Jerome J. Schulte et al., "You're the Flight Surgeon. Anxiety," *Aviation, Space, and Environmental Medicine* 74, no. 8 (2003): 894–895.
6. A. Quesnot and A. Alperovitch, "Snoring and Risk of Cognitive Decline: A 4-Year Follow-Up Study in 1389 Older Individuals," *Journal of the American Geriatrics Society* 47, no. 9 (1999): 1159–1160.
7. J. H. Ficker et al., "Are Snoring Medical Students at Risk of Failing Their Exams?" *Sleep* 22, no. 2 (1999): 205–209.
8. K. A. Franklin et al., "Snoring, Pregnancy-Induced Hypertension, and Growth Retardation of the Fetus," *Chest Journal* 117, no. 1 (2000): 137–141.
9. F. B. Hu et al., Snoring and Risk of Cardiovascular Disease in Women," *Journal of the American College of Cardiology* 35, no. 2 (2000): 308–313.
10. Wael K. Al-Delaimy et al., "Snoring as a Risk Factor for Type II Diabetes Mellitus: A Prospective Study," *American Journal of Epidemiology* 155, no. 5 (2002): 387–393.
11. Augusto Zaninelli et al., "Snoring and Risk of Cardiovascular Disease," *International Journal of Cardiology* 32, no. 3 (1991): 347–351.
12. Ravi Kanagala et al., "Obstructive Sleep Apnea and the Recurrence of Atrial Fibrillation," *Circulation* 107, no. 20 (2003): 2589–2594.
13. P.A. Lafranchi et al., "Prognostic Value of Nocturnal Cheyne-Stokes Respiration in Chronic Heart Failure," *Circulation* 99, no. 11 (1999): 1435–1440.
14. Paul E. Peppard et al., "Prospective Study of the Association Between Sleep-Disordered Breathing and Hypertension," *New England Journal of Medicine* 342, no. 19 (2000): 1378–1384.
15. Rainier Dziewas et al., "Increased Prevalence of Sleep Apnea in Patients with Recurring Ischemic Stroke Compared with First Stroke Victims," *Journal of Neurology* 252, no. 11 (2005): 1394–1398.
16. Apoor S. Gami et al., "Familial Premature Coronary Artery Disease Mortality and Obstructive Sleep Apnea," *Chest Journal* 131, no. 1 (2007): 118–121.
17. Olivier Milleron et al., "Benefits of Obstructive Sleep Apnoea Treatment in Coronary Artery Disease: A Long-Term Follow-Up Study," *European Heart Journal* 25, no. 9 (2004): 728–734.
18. Colin E. Sullivan et al., "Reversal of Obstructive Sleep Apnea by Continuous Positive Airway Pressure Applied Through the Nares," *Lancet* 317, no. 8225 (1981): 862–865.
19. Markku Partinen et al., "Long-term Outcome for Obstructive Sleep Apnea Syndrome Patients," *Chest Journal* 94, no. 6 (1998):1200–1204.
20. T. Douglas Bradley et al., "Continuous Positive Airway Pressure for Central Sleep Apnea and Heart Failure," *New England Journal of Medicine* 35, no. 19 (2005): 2025–2033.

21. Philippe Jaoude et al., "Survival Benefit of CPAP Favors Hypercapnic Patients with the Overlap Syndrome," *Lung* 192 (2014): 251–258.

About the Author

Doctor Fisher lives in Los Angeles with his partner Judith Pacht; their four children are scattered across the US and the UK. By the end of his formal education he had become a physician. After residency and subspecialty training, he became a board-certified specialist of Sleep Medicine, Pulmonary Diseases and Internal Medicine. His private practice continued for forty years, until he retired several years ago from patient care and as Clinical Professor of Medicine at UCLA. He now especially enjoys tennis and photography.

Sleep: A User's Guide is his first full length book, although he previously wrote (with the late Myron Stein MD) a booklet for patients with asthma at the request of the American College of Chest Physicians. He has authored more than twenty medical research papers. He has contributed chapters to books published by UCLA and the Fogarty Center of the National Institutes of Health, and has written articles for local newspapers. A popular lecturer, he has given hundreds of talks to audiences of the general public as well as to physicians at every level of training and practice, and has been invited to comment on public health issues for TV news programs in Los Angeles.

Connect with him online at hkennethfisher.com and on social media @SleepAUsersGuide.

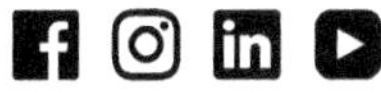

www.ingramcontent.com/pod-product-compliance
Lightning Source LLC
Chambersburg PA
CBHW052134270326
41930CB00012B/2874
* 9 7 8 1 6 1 1 5 3 5 8 0 8 *